# Psychedelic Therapeutics: A Comprehensive Guide to MDMA

**Psychedelic Therapeutics Series, Volume 3**

Dr. Nikolaos Tsilikas

Published by Nikolaos Tsilikas, 2025.

PSYCHEDELIC THERAPEUTICS: A COMPREHENSIVE GUIDE TO MDMA

**First edition. February 3, 2025.**



ISBN: 979-8227426253

Written by Dr. Nikolaos Tsilikas.

# Table of Contents

# Chapter 1. Why MDMA and Why Now?

Welcome to the third installment of the *Psychedelic Therapeutics Series*. Following the rapid success of the first two volumes—focused on psilocybin and LSD—this new book turns its attention to an equally compelling yet distinct agent: MDMA (3,4-methylenedioxymethamphetamine). Historically caricatured as a mere "party drug," MDMA has recently garnered scientific acclaim for its remarkable efficacy in treating mental health conditions that often resist conventional therapies (Carhart-Harris & Goodwin, 2017; Mithoefer et al., 2019).

Like its predecessors, this volume aims to bridge rigorous scientific research with clinical practice. The evolution in how we perceive MDMA, much like the shifts witnessed with psilocybin and LSD, underscores a broader renaissance in psychedelic and empathogenic medicine—one that seeks innovative, evidence-based methods to address conditions such as post-traumatic stress disorder (PTSD), social anxiety, and treatment-resistant depression (Sessa, 2017; Tupper et al., 2015).

By retracing MDMA's journey from pharmaceutical obscurity and underground use to "breakthrough therapy" status, we will explore its unique neurochemical and psychological properties, as well as the regulatory landscape that shapes its clinical future. This chapter lays out the central themes that will guide the discussion, highlighting both the immense therapeutic potential of MDMA and the ethical, legal, and practical considerations that accompany its resurgent prominence (Jerome et al., 2020).

## 1.1 Background of Renewed Interest

In order to grasp why MDMA is now poised for a transformative role in psychiatry, one must appreciate the broader context of the psychedelic renaissance. Over the past two decades, researchers have revisited substances long sidelined by legal and cultural barriers, demonstrating significant therapeutic benefits in controlled settings (Carhart-Harris & Goodwin, 2017). Against this backdrop, MDMA emerges not as a classical psychedelic, but as a unique empathogen—fostering emotional openness and attenuating fear responses without inducing the visual or auditory hallucinations characteristic of LSD or psilocybin (Nichols, 2016).

## The Psychedelic Renaissance

The term "psychedelic renaissance" refers to a revival of scientific and clinical interest in psychoactive compounds once considered taboo in mainstream research (Tupper et al., 2015). While psilocybin and LSD have led much of this renewed curiosity—showing promise in treating depression, anxiety, addiction, and existential distress—MDMA's capacity to facilitate trust and empathy has now taken center stage, particularly in the realm of trauma-focused psychotherapy (Sessa, 2017).

## MDMA vs. Classical Psychedelics

Despite being grouped with psychedelics in popular discourse, MDMA differs markedly in both pharmacological action and subjective experience (Bedi et al., 2009; Nichols, 2016). Classical psychedelics often precipitate ego-dissolving or highly introspective states linked to serotonin 5-HT2A receptor agonism, whereas MDMA's distinct profile includes robust increases in serotonin, dopamine, and norepinephrine (Baggott, 2016; Mithoefer et al., 2019). This biochemical interplay yields empathogenic effects—enhanced emotional warmth, lowered defensive barriers, and a willingness to engage deeply with painful or traumatic memories (Jerome et al., 2020).

## Therapeutic Breakthroughs

A defining moment in MDMA's modern narrative arrived when the U.S. Food and Drug Administration granted it "breakthrough therapy" designation for PTSD (Feduccia & Mithoefer, 2018). This regulatory milestone was based on compelling data from clinical trials, particularly those spearheaded by the Multidisciplinary Association for Psychedelic Studies (MAPS). Early phase studies have demonstrated substantial alleviation of PTSD symptoms in participants who previously struggled to find relief through conventional treatments (Mithoefer et al., 2019).

These promising outcomes are fueling an acceleration of clinical research, paralleled by shifts in public opinion and policy. As with psilocybin and LSD,

MDMA's reemergence underscores a changing landscape in mental health care, where deeply ingrained stigmas are giving way to nuanced, evidence-based evaluations of novel treatments.

## Conclusion

MDMA's resurgence is emblematic of a broader reevaluation of psychedelics in contemporary medicine. Grounded in both rigorous research and a shifting cultural paradigm, this empathogen stands poised to offer breakthroughs in the treatment of PTSD, anxiety, and beyond. The following chapters will delve deeper into MDMA's rich history, pharmacological underpinnings, clinical applications, and the regulatory developments shaping its future. By integrating scientific rigor with open-minded exploration—much like the approach used in our volumes on psilocybin and LSD—this book seeks to provide a comprehensive guide to one of the most intriguing and potentially transformative agents in modern psychiatric practice.

---

## References


- Baggott, M. J. (2016). What do we know about MDMA's mechanism of action? Mechanistic and methodological considerations. AAPS Journal, 18(5), 1139–1159.
- Bedi, G., Hyman, D., & de Wit, H. (2009). Is ecstasy an "empathogen"? Effects of ±3,4-methylenedioxymethamphetamine on prosocial feelings and identification of emotional states in others. Biological Psychiatry, 65(10), 722–727.
- Carhart-Harris, R. L., & Goodwin, G. M. (2017). The therapeutic potential of psychedelic drugs: Past, present, and future. Neuropsychopharmacology, 42(11), 2105–2113.
- Feduccia, A. A., & Mithoefer, M. C. (2018). MDMA-assisted psychotherapy for PTSD: Are memory reconsolidation and fear extinction underlying mechanisms? Progress in Neuro-Psychopharmacology & Biological Psychiatry, 84(Pt B), 221–228.
- Jerome, I., Feduccia, A. A., & Mithoefer, M. (2020). MDMA-assisted psychotherapy for the treatment of posttraumatic stress disorder:

What do we know and what comes next? Current Psychiatry Reports, 22(5), 25.

- Mithoefer, M. C., Mithoefer, A. T., Jerome, I., et al. (2019). 3,4-Methylenedioxymethamphetamine (MDMA)-assisted psychotherapy for posttraumatic stress disorder in military veterans, firefighters, and police officers. Journal of Psychopharmacology, 33(9), 1054–1067.
- Nichols, D. E. (2016). Psychedelics. Pharmacological Reviews, 68(2), 264–355.
- Sessa, B. (2017). MDMA and PTSD treatment: "PTSD: From novel pathophysiology to innovative therapeutics." Neuroscience Letters, 649, 176–180.
- Tupper, K. W., Wood, E., Yensen, R., & Johnson, M. W. (2015). Psychedelic medicine: A re-emerging therapeutic paradigm. CMAJ, 187(14), 1054–1059.

## 1.2 Overview of This Volume

A comprehensive exploration of MDMA requires an interdisciplinary lens that encompasses its history, pharmacology, therapeutic framework, and evolving role in modern psychiatry. In this volume, readers will encounter both the scientific rigor that underpins MDMA-assisted therapy and the nuanced ethical considerations involved in bringing a once-stigmatized substance into mainstream treatment (Mithoefer et al., 2019; Sessa, 2017). The chapters to follow aim to provide a balanced perspective—addressing promising clinical outcomes, potential risks, and the broader cultural contexts that shape MDMA's status today.

---

### Key Themes and Organization

**The Therapeutic Arc of MDMA**

Unlike classical psychedelics such as psilocybin or LSD, MDMA does not typically induce pronounced hallucinations (Nichols, 2016). Instead, it facilitates a state of heightened empathy, emotional openness, and reduced fear responses, making it particularly suited for trauma-focused psychotherapy (Sessa, 2017; Doblin et al., 2019). This unique psychoactive profile is explored in depth across multiple chapters, beginning with a historical overview and culminating in future-oriented discussions about research expansions and policy reform.

**Safety, Efficacy, and Clinical Frameworks**

Building on the foundational research conducted by organizations like the Multidisciplinary Association for Psychedelic Studies (MAPS), this volume examines MDMA's safety profile, pharmacological nuances, and clinical efficacy (Mithoefer et al., 2019). Detailed attention is given to the structured protocols that define MDMA-assisted psychotherapy—spanning patient selection, session design, and post-experience integration (Jerome et al., 2020). By highlighting evidence-based practices, the aim is to empower psychiatrists, therapists, and researchers with actionable guidelines that prioritize patient well-being.

---

## Bridging Science and Psychiatry

### Evidence Synthesis and Ethical Considerations

A central ambition of this book is to bridge rigorous scientific inquiry with the evolving needs of modern mental health care (Carhart-Harris & Goodwin, 2017). Although MDMA enjoys "breakthrough therapy" designation by the FDA for post-traumatic stress disorder (PTSD), questions remain regarding broader clinical applications, such as depression, social anxiety, and addiction (Sessa, 2017; Jerome et al., 2020). Chapters dedicated to ethical and practical concerns underscore the importance of informed consent, medical screening, and expert supervision. These elements collectively form the cornerstone of responsible MDMA-assisted therapy, positioning the substance as a complement—rather than a replacement—to established mental health interventions.

### Intersection with Cultural Shifts

MDMA's trajectory from "party drug" to potential psychiatric tool reflects shifting cultural and political landscapes (Doblin et al., 2019). This volume recognizes that effective clinical adoption must consider broader societal contexts, including changing public perceptions, legal reform efforts, and the role of advocacy groups. By discussing these cultural dimensions alongside clinical findings, the book aims to offer a holistic view of MDMA's current and future place in psychiatry.

## What to Expect

### Practical and Evidence-Based Guidance

Clinicians, researchers, and interested readers will find a structured road map for understanding and integrating MDMA into therapeutic practice (Mithoefer et al., 2019). This includes detailed descriptions of session models—covering dosing protocols, set and setting considerations, and outcome measures. Additionally, case studies and personal vignettes provide real-world examples that highlight both the transformative potential and the inherent complexities of MDMA-assisted therapy (Jerome et al., 2020).

### A Launching Point for Ongoing Inquiry

Finally, this volume serves as a catalyst for further investigation. While MDMA's efficacy for PTSD is well-documented, emerging research explores its promise in other domains—such as depression, couples therapy, and end-of-life anxiety (Sessa, 2017). By the conclusion of this book, readers will be equipped with an analytical framework that fosters deeper engagement with MDMA's evolving research base, regulatory pathways, and therapeutic frontiers (Doblin et al., 2019).

## References


- Carhart-Harris, R. L., & Goodwin, G. M. (2017). The therapeutic potential of psychedelic drugs: Past, present, and future. *Neuropsychopharmacology, 42*(11), 2105–2113.
- Doblin, R. E., Christiansen, M., Jerome, I., & Burge, B. (2019). The past and future of MDMA-assisted psychotherapy for PTSD. *Journal of Psychopharmacology, 33*(10), 1180–1187.
- Jerome, I., Feduccia, A. A., & Mithoefer, M. C. (2020). MDMA-assisted psychotherapy and its role in the treatment of PTSD. *Frontiers in Psychiatry, 11*, 562114.
- Mithoefer, M. C., Feduccia, A. A., Jerome, I., et al. (2019). MDMA-assisted psychotherapy for treatment of PTSD: Study of safety and efficacy. *Journal of Psychopharmacology, 33*(10), 1141–1151.
- Nichols, D. E. (2016). Psychedelics. *Pharmacological Reviews, 68*(2), 264–355.
- Sessa, B. (2017). MDMA and LSD in the treatment of PTSD, anxiety, and addiction: A narrative review. *Journal of Psychoactive Drugs, 49*(3), 212–220.

## 1.3 The Role of MDMA in Modern Psychiatry

Understanding MDMA's position in contemporary mental health care requires a nuanced examination of its unique pharmacological properties, emerging therapeutic evidence, and evolving cultural acceptance. While traditional treatments for conditions such as posttraumatic stress disorder (PTSD), depression, and social anxiety have relied primarily on pharmacological agents that suppress or modulate symptoms, MDMA-assisted psychotherapy focuses on enhancing emotional openness, reducing fear responses, and facilitating introspective breakthroughs (Mithoefer et al., 2019; Sessa, 2017). This section explores how MDMA is reshaping psychiatric approaches to trauma, aiding in other treatment-resistant conditions, and catalyzing broader policy shifts that may usher in a new era of integrative mental health interventions.

### Revolutionizing Trauma Therapy

MDMA's most prominent role in modern psychiatry has emerged in the treatment of PTSD (Mithoefer et al., 2019). In contrast to selective serotonin reuptake inhibitors (SSRIs), which can blunt emotional responsiveness, MDMA appears to help patients face and process traumatic memories without becoming overwhelmed by fear. Its capacity to temporarily reduce amygdala hyperactivity allows for deeper engagement with trauma-related content, creating conditions in which patients can revisit painful experiences with a heightened sense of safety (Jerome et al., 2020).

When administered under clinical supervision, MDMA-assisted psychotherapy typically involves structured preparation, controlled dosing, and post-session integration work. Therapists report that participants are more receptive to discussing emotionally charged topics, enabling them to access insights that might remain unreachable under conventional therapeutic modalities (Greer & Tolbert, 1986). These observations, buttressed by rigorous clinical trials, have positioned MDMA as a "breakthrough therapy" for PTSD, reflecting a paradigm shift in how trauma can be approached and potentially resolved in psychiatric settings (Mithoefer et al., 2019).

## Beyond PTSD: Expanding Psychiatric Applications

While PTSD remains the primary focus of MDMA research, emerging data suggest a broader therapeutic potential. Ongoing studies are evaluating MDMA for depression, anxiety disorders, and other psychiatric conditions that resist conventional treatment (Sessa, 2017). One particularly notable pilot study used MDMA-assisted psychotherapy to reduce social anxiety in adults on the autism spectrum (Danforth et al., 2016). Participants reported a greater ability to understand and communicate emotions, bolstering the theory that MDMA facilitates pro-social behavior by amplifying empathy and positive affect (Hysek et al., 2012).

Additionally, anecdotal reports and preliminary trials hint at MDMA's usefulness in couples therapy, where entrenched relational conflicts might be navigated more effectively under the drug's prosocial influence (Greer & Tolbert, 1986). Although research in these areas is nascent, the potential scope of MDMA's clinical relevance extends beyond trauma-specific syndromes, prompting further exploration into how emotional openness might transform other facets of psychiatric care.

## Shifting Cultural and Legal Perspectives

MDMA's evolving reputation—from a prohibited "party drug" to a possible cornerstone of psychiatric practice—reflects broader cultural and regulatory shifts (Carhart-Harris & Nutt, 2017). In the United States, Phase 3 trials sponsored by organizations like the Multidisciplinary Association for Psychedelic Studies (MAPS) have garnered "breakthrough therapy" status by the FDA, expediting research timelines and raising public awareness (Jerome et al., 2020). Similar developments in Canada, Australia, and parts of Europe underscore a growing consensus that MDMA, when administered responsibly, holds promise for legitimizing new therapeutic frameworks.

This transformation has not been without challenges. Concerns about abuse potential, neurotoxicity, and the broader social implications of expanding legal access persist (Sessa, 2017). Nevertheless, the momentum behind MDMA research—driven by promising clinical data and increasing societal openness to psychedelic therapies—has prompted policymakers to reassess the risk-benefit balance, paving the way for expanded studies and, potentially, mainstream adoption (Mithoefer et al., 2019).

## Conclusion

MDMA's resurgence in psychiatry illustrates the shifting priorities of a field now more willing to integrate novel therapies that foster emotional processing, introspection, and personal growth. Its application in PTSD stands as the strongest evidence base, but nascent research on social anxiety, depression, and even couples therapy suggests that MDMA's impact could be significantly broader. As legislative barriers continue to recede, future studies will clarify its full therapeutic range, optimal treatment protocols, and long-term safety profile (Danforth et al., 2016; Jerome et al., 2020). In an era increasingly defined by complex mental health challenges, MDMA represents both a promising clinical tool and a catalyst for reimagining how psychiatry addresses the emotional core of psychological distress.

## References


- Carhart-Harris, R. L., & Nutt, D. J. (2017). Serotonin and brain function: A tale of two receptors. *Journal of Psychopharmacology, 31*(9), 1091–1120.
- Danforth, A. L., Grob, C. S., Struble, C. M., et al. (2016). Reduction in social anxiety after MDMA-assisted psychotherapy with autistic adults: A randomized, double-blind, placebo-controlled pilot study. *Psychopharmacology, 233*(6), 1033–1042.
- Greer, G., & Tolbert, R. (1986). Subjective reports of the effects of MDMA in a clinical setting. *Journal of Psychoactive Drugs, 18*(4), 319–327.
- Hysek, C. M., Domes, G., & Liechti, M. E. (2012). MDMA enhances "mind reading" of positive emotions and impairs "mind reading" of negative emotions. *Psychopharmacology, 222*(2), 293–302.
- Jerome, L., Schuster, S., et al. (2020). Long-term follow-up outcomes of MDMA-assisted psychotherapy for PTSD. *European Journal of*

*Psychotraumatology, 11*(1), 1708343.

- Mithoefer, M. C., Feduccia, A. A., Jerome, L., et al. (2019). MDMA-assisted psychotherapy for posttraumatic stress disorder: A systematic review of modern clinical studies. *Journal of Psychopharmacology, 33*(9), 1088–1102.
- Sessa, B. (2017). MDMA therapy for PTSD and beyond. *The British Journal of Psychiatry, 210*(2), 9–11.

# Chapter 2. Historical and Cultural Context

MDMA's journey from a little-known chemical compound to a pivotal subject of modern psychiatric research is marked by sharp contrasts between its therapeutic promise and its period of criminalization. This chapter explores the interplay of scientific innovation, cultural shifts, and political decisions that shaped MDMA's complex reputation.

Early references to MDMA emerged in pharmaceutical archives dating back to 1912, yet it remained in obscurity until the mid-to-late 20th century (Passie & Benzenhöfer, 2018). As word of its unique psychoactive properties spread, various psychiatrists and therapists began investigating its therapeutic utility—particularly its ability to facilitate emotional openness. However, rising concerns over recreational misuse in the 1980s led to global prohibition efforts. Understanding this historical and cultural background is essential for appreciating why contemporary research into MDMA faces both enthusiasm and regulatory barriers.

## 2.1 Discovery and Early Use

In contrast to many classical psychedelics that emerged from ethnobotanical traditions, MDMA was a laboratory synthesis. While its empathogenic properties would later garner attention, the compound's origins began in the realm of pharmaceutical research and largely went unnoticed for decades.

### Initial Synthesis and Patent by Merck

- **1912: Accidental Discovery**
  MDMA (3,4-Methylenedioxymethamphetamine) was first synthesized by chemists at the German pharmaceutical company Merck, reportedly while attempting to develop a hemostatic agent (Benzenhöfer & Passie, 2010). Merck patented the compound in 1914, but no significant medical use was pursued at the time (Freudenmann et al., 2006).
- **Dormancy in Early Records**

After its initial documentation, MDMA remained largely dormant for many decades. Compared to other synthesized compounds of the period, it did not attract clinical or commercial interest (Passie & Benzenhöfer, 2018). Consequently, historical references to MDMA between 1912 and the 1950s are scarce, reflecting the compound's peripheral status during that era.

## Rediscovery by Alexander Shulgin

- **1970s: Renewed Attention**
  Renowned chemist Alexander "Sasha" Shulgin introduced MDMA into scientific and therapeutic discourse in the 1970s. Intrigued by its empathogenic qualities, Shulgin synthesized MDMA anew and shared samples with a network of psychotherapists (Shulgin & Shulgin, 1991). During informal sessions, clinicians observed enhanced emotional transparency and reduced fear responses in patients—a stark contrast to the ego dissolution commonly reported with classical psychedelics like LSD or psilocybin.
- **Shulgin's Role in Empathogen Research**
  Shulgin's systematic approach to psychoactive compounds paved the way for an emerging class of "entactogens" or "empathogens," which included MDMA (Nichols, 1986). By meticulously documenting qualitative effects, Shulgin elevated MDMA from obscurity to a compound of significant interest among select circles of therapists, ultimately sparking broader conversations on its clinical potential.

## Therapeutic Uses in the 1970s and Early 1980s

- **Experimental Psychotherapy Sessions**
  Psychotherapists, primarily in the United States, began using MDMA for couples therapy, anxiety-related disorders, and trauma processing in the late 1970s and early 1980s (Greer & Tolbert, 1986). Clinicians reported that MDMA facilitated trust and emotional openness, helping patients confront and articulate distressing

experiences without the intense fear responses they might otherwise experience.

- **Emergent Clinical Observations**
  Although these early sessions were not part of large-scale clinical trials, anecdotal reports suggested potential benefits:
    - **Reduced Emotional Defensiveness** – Patients seemed more willing to explore painful memories (Greer & Tolbert, 1986).
    - **Strengthened Therapeutic Alliance** – Therapists noted that MDMA sessions often deepened rapport, enabling more honest communication (Stolaroff, 2004).

## Setting the Stage for Future Debates

During this period, MDMA existed in a legal grey area, as regulatory agencies had yet to recognize it as a distinct substance requiring control (Freudenmann et al., 2006). However, growing recreational use and media attention in the early 1980s foreshadowed the intensifying debates that would soon envelop MDMA. The stage was set for an inevitable clash between its promising therapeutic applications and rising concerns regarding non-medical misuse.

## References


- Benzenhöfer, U., & Passie, T. (2010). Rediscovering MDMA (Ecstasy): The role of the American chemist Alexander T. Shulgin. Addiction, 105(8), 1355–1361.
- Freudenmann, R. W., Öxler, F., & Bernschneider-Reif, S. (2006). The origin of MDMA (ecstasy) revisited: The true story reconstructed from the original documents. Addiction, 101(9), 1241–1245.
- Greer, G., & Tolbert, R. (1986). Subjective reports of the effects of MDMA in a clinical setting. Journal of Psychoactive Drugs, 18(4), 319–327.
- Nichols, D. E. (1986). Differences between the mechanism of action of MDMA, MBDB, and the classic hallucinogens. Journal of Psychoactive Drugs, 18(4), 305–313.
- Passie, T., & Benzenhöfer, U. (2018). The early history of 'Ecstasy'.

Neuropathics & Psychoactive Substances, 7(2), 181–189.
- Shulgin, A. T., & Shulgin, A. (1991). PIHKAL: A Chemical Love Story. Transform Press.
- Stolaroff, M. J. (2004). The secret chief revealed: Conversations with a pioneer of the underground therapy movement. MAPS Bulletin, 14(2), 15–22.

## 2.2 MDMA in Psychotherapy Before Prohibition

Before MDMA's eventual classification as a Schedule I substance in 1985, a small yet dedicated community of therapists and researchers explored its potential for treating a range of psychological issues. Far from the realm of nightlife and recreational "Ecstasy" use, these early practitioners approached MDMA as a novel tool for deep emotional processing, relationship counseling, and trauma resolution (Greer & Tolbert, 1986; Adamson & Metzner, 1988). This chapter provides a detailed examination of MDMA's emergence in psychotherapy prior to its criminalization, highlighting the key figures, reported therapeutic effects, and factors that ultimately led to its prohibition.

### Early Adoption by Psychotherapists

#### Discovery and Rediscovery

Although MDMA was first synthesized by Merck in 1912, it remained virtually unknown in clinical settings until the 1970s, when chemist Alexander Shulgin synthesized and self-tested the substance, noting its unique psycho-empathic effects (Shulgin & Nichols, 1978; Shulgin & Shulgin, 1991). Enthralled by its capacity to reduce fear and enhance openness, Shulgin introduced MDMA to select therapists who were active in the psychedelic research community.

#### Therapeutic Circles

Psychologists and psychiatrists who had previously worked with other psychedelics—most notably LSD—were drawn to MDMA's capacity for facilitating emotional intimacy without the more disorienting perceptual distortions often seen with classic hallucinogens (Greer & Tolbert, 1986). Early adopters reported that patients could confront difficult emotions and memories with reduced anxiety, fostering more direct and compassionate engagement with core psychological issues (Adamson & Metzner, 1988).

### Reported Benefits in Clinical and Relational Contexts

#### Enhanced Emotional Clarity

One of the recurring themes in these early, semi-underground clinical sessions was MDMA's ability to facilitate emotional clarity and empathetic communication. Patients described feeling deeply connected to themselves and others, which proved especially valuable in couples therapy and family counseling contexts (Greer & Tolbert, 1986). Therapists noted that individuals seemed more willing to discuss sensitive personal topics, accelerating progress that might have otherwise taken months in standard talk therapy.

**Reduction in Defensive Barriers**

MDMA's influence on serotonin and other neurotransmitters appeared to temporarily lower psychological defenses, allowing repressed memories and emotions to surface in a controlled manner (Shulgin & Shulgin, 1991). Early case reports detailed patients who could safely revisit traumatic experiences with significantly less terror, a phenomenon later corroborated by more formalized research into MDMA-assisted therapy for PTSD (Greer & Tolbert, 1990; Mithoefer et al., 2010).

**Integrative Follow-Up**

While many of these sessions were relatively short (ranging from a few hours to a full day), the aftereffects often lingered as patients integrated insights into their daily lives (Adamson & Metzner, 1988). Similar to observations seen with classic psychedelics, a substantial emphasis was placed on "integration" sessions, wherein therapists helped individuals process revelations from the MDMA experience and adapt their new perspectives into behavioral change.

## Transition to Criminalization

### Growing Popularity and Concern

As the positive reports spread informally among therapists, MDMA also began appearing in recreational settings under the street name "Ecstasy." Its rising popularity caught the attention of U.S. authorities, who became concerned about its non-medical consumption and potential for misuse (Shulgin & Nichols, 1978; Peroutka, 1987). Despite objections from many therapists already utilizing MDMA with promising outcomes, the Drug Enforcement Administration (DEA) moved toward scheduling the substance.

**DEA Scheduling and the End of an Era**

In 1985, the DEA classified MDMA as a Schedule I drug—defined as having "no accepted medical use and a high potential for abuse" (Doblin, 2002). This legal action effectively halted formal clinical investigations, pushed MDMA-assisted therapy underground, and stymied what many researchers believed was a potentially game-changing development in psychotherapy (Greer & Tolbert, 1990).

## Conclusion

Prior to its prohibition, MDMA occupied a unique niche in psychotherapy, offering a gentler alternative to classic psychedelics and enabling profound emotional processing in a relatively short span of time (Adamson & Metzner, 1988). Early therapists working with MDMA reported encouraging results across a range of psychological and relational challenges, yet the drug's swift move into the recreational scene and subsequent legal restrictions curtailed this promising research. Although the early momentum was disrupted, the insights gleaned during this period laid the groundwork for the modern resurgence of interest in MDMA-assisted therapy—a development that would eventually gain formal traction decades later.

## References


- Adamson, S., & Metzner, R. (1988). The nature of the MDMA experience and its role in healing, psychotherapy, and spiritual practice. *ReVision*, 10(4), 59–72.
- Doblin, R. (2002). A clinical plan for MDMA (ecstasy) in the treatment of posttraumatic stress disorder (PTSD): Partnering with the FDA. *Journal of Psychoactive Drugs*, 34(2), 185–194.
- Greer, G., & Tolbert, R. (1986). Subjective reports of the effects of MDMA in a clinical setting. *Journal of Psychoactive Drugs*, 18(4), 319–327.
- Greer, G., & Tolbert, R. (1990). The therapeutic use of MDMA. In S. J. Satel (Ed.), *Drug abuse and social policy* (pp. 465–476). U.S. Government Printing Office.
- Mithoefer, M. C., Wagner, M., Mithoefer, A. T., et al. (2010). The

safety and efficacy of ±3,4-methylenedioxymethamphetamine-assisted psychotherapy in subjects with chronic, treatment-resistant posttraumatic stress disorder: The first randomized controlled pilot study. *Journal of Psychopharmacology*, 25(4), 439–452.

- Peroutka, S. J. (1987). Incidence of recreational use of MDMA (ecstasy) on an undergraduate campus. *New England Journal of Medicine*, 317(26), 1542.
- Shulgin, A. T., & Nichols, D. E. (1978). Characterization of three new psychotomimetics. *In Proceedings of the 1978 National Conference on the Psychopharmacology of Hallucinogens* (pp. 65–72). National Institute of Mental Health.
- Shulgin, A. T., & Shulgin, A. (1991). *Pihkal: A chemical love story.* Transform Press.

## 2.3 The Criminalization and Illicit Use Era

In tracing the trajectory of MDMA from a quietly used psychotherapeutic adjunct to a widely recognized club drug, it is crucial to understand the socio-political context that led to its prohibition. This chapter examines the surge in non-clinical use of MDMA in the early 1980s, the subsequent governmental response, and the far-reaching impact of Schedule I classification on both cultural attitudes and scientific progress (Beck & Rosenbaum, 1994; Freedman, 1985).

### Escalation of MDMA Use in Recreational Settings

#### Early Recreational Popularity

By the late 1970s, MDMA had begun to spread beyond the small therapeutic circles that had quietly explored its potential for trauma and couples counseling (Doblin, 2002). Users in dance clubs and communal gatherings found MDMA's empathogenic qualities—its capacity to induce euphoria, empathy, and heightened sociability—uniquely suited to fostering a sense of collective "togetherness" (Beck & Rosenbaum, 1994). Its newfound popularity in these social arenas quickly outpaced the measured, clinical-style use observed in early psychotherapy.

#### Rise of "Ecstasy"

As recreational demand soared, entrepreneurs and illicit chemists rebranded MDMA under the moniker "Ecstasy." While early formulations were often relatively pure, varying sources and illegal manufacturing led to inconsistent products (National Institute on Drug Abuse, 2020). This variability introduced health risks and fueled sensational media reports, laying the groundwork for a robust public outcry.

### Government Action and Scheduling

#### DEA Emergency Scheduling

A pivotal moment came in 1985, when the U.S. Drug Enforcement Administration (DEA) invoked its emergency scheduling authority to classify MDMA as a Schedule I substance, effectively criminalizing its manufacture, distribution, and use (Freedman, 1985). This decision was controversial, as many therapists and researchers who had witnessed MDMA's therapeutic benefits argued for a more nuanced regulatory approach. Nonetheless, concerns about rising recreational misuse, potential neurotoxicity, and moral panic drove the U.S. government to enact strict prohibition (Sessa, 2017).

**International Ripple Effects**

Following the U.S. lead, other nations, including Canada, Australia, and many European countries, quickly introduced similar bans (National Institute on Drug Abuse, 2020). Within a few short years, MDMA transitioned from an obscure therapeutic adjunct to one of the most heavily scrutinized and policed substances worldwide. This swift, near-global criminalization fractured ongoing research efforts, leaving many promising clinical inquiries at a standstill (Doblin, 2002).

## Impact on Research and Public Perception

### Halted Scientific Progress

Criminalization profoundly constrained formal research on MDMA's potential benefits. Until the 2010s, the majority of sanctioned studies were limited to animal models assessing potential harm rather than human trials exploring therapeutic efficacy (Sessa, 2017). Institutional review boards, already wary of psychedelic research, faced additional layers of regulatory and funding barriers. Consequently, many of the positive anecdotal and early clinical reports from psychotherapists remained unpublished or relegated to underground literature.

**Stigmatization and Misinformation**

Public perception of MDMA became dominated by cautionary tales of "brain damage" and sensational media stories linking Ecstasy to fatal overdoses (Freedman, 1985; National Institute on Drug Abuse, 2020). While impurities and adulterants in illicitly manufactured tablets significantly contributed to adverse outcomes, these nuances were lost in mainstream narratives that conflated all forms of MDMA with dangerous hedonism. This stigmatization persisted for decades, marginalizing advocates who sought to explore MDMA's therapeutic potential (Beck & Rosenbaum, 1994).

## The Underground Therapeutic Community

### Continued Unofficial Use

Despite prohibition, a small but dedicated network of underground therapists persisted in using MDMA for psychological healing (Doblin, 2002). Often operating in legal gray zones or entirely outside regulatory frameworks, these practitioners believed that MDMA's empathogenic effects uniquely supported trauma processing and interpersonal breakthroughs. While these unsanctioned efforts generated compelling anecdotal testimonials, the lack of official oversight and peer-reviewed publications limited their broader impact.

### Catalyst for Future Reappraisal

The underground community's experiences would later inform organizations like the Multidisciplinary Association for Psychedelic Studies (MAPS), which spearheaded formal clinical trials in collaboration with regulatory agencies. Although criminalization created formidable barriers, it also spurred a grassroots movement that preserved MDMA's therapeutic legacy until the climate was ripe for renewed scientific inquiry (Sessa, 2017).

## Conclusion

The criminalization of MDMA in the mid-1980s not only curtailed its legal therapeutic use but also accelerated its entrenchment in recreational subcultures. Despite legitimate concerns about substance misuse, the abrupt prohibition often conflated clinical potential with illegal hedonism, thereby stalling research for nearly two decades (Freedman, 1985; National Institute on Drug Abuse, 2020). Yet, in the shadows of legal restrictions, a quiet but determined underground community sustained interest in MDMA's healing properties. This dichotomy set the stage for the eventual resurgence of formal research, now poised to reshape both medical practice and public perception of the drug (Doblin, 2002; Sessa, 2017).

## References


- Beck, J., & Rosenbaum, M. (1994). *Pursuit of Ecstasy: The MDMA Experience*. SUNY Press.
- Doblin, R. (2002). A clinical plan for MDMA (Ecstasy) in the US.

*MAPS Bulletin*, 12(2), 3–7.

- Freedman, R. (1985). Scheduling of MDMA: The debate and implications. *Journal of Psychoactive Drugs*, 17(2), 115–121.
- National Institute on Drug Abuse. (2020). *MDMA (Ecstasy/Molly) DrugFacts*. Retrieved from https://nida.nih.gov
- Sessa, B. (2017). MDMA therapy: A new treatment model for PTSD and beyond. *Neurotherapeutics*, 14(3), 554–560.

# Chapter 3. Pharmacology and Neuroscience of MDMA

The pharmacological profile of 3,4-methylenedioxymethamphetamine (MDMA) sets it apart from both classical psychedelics (e.g., LSD, psilocybin) and traditional stimulants (e.g., amphetamine, methamphetamine). Although MDMA does share certain chemical similarities with amphetamines, its empathogenic properties—characterized by heightened emotional openness and empathy—emerge through a unique blend of serotonergic, dopaminergic, and noradrenergic effects (Nichols, 1986; Green et al., 2003). This chapter explores the distinct chemical structure of MDMA, its underlying mechanism of action, and the broader neurological processes that account for its therapeutic potential and associated risks.

## 3.1 Chemical Structure and Mechanism of Action

In examining MDMA's pharmacology, it is essential to highlight the structural features and receptor interactions that differentiate this compound from both classic psychedelics and purely stimulant agents. While classical psychedelics primarily target serotonin 2A (5-HT2A) receptors to induce hallucinogenic states, MDMA acts as a releasing agent and reuptake inhibitor of monoamines—particularly serotonin (5-HT), but also dopamine (DA) and norepinephrine (NE)—thereby fostering a unique psycho-emotional state often referred to as "empathogenic" or "entactogenic" (Nichols, 1986; Liechti & Vollenweider, 2001).

### Structural Overview

Chemically, MDMA belongs to the substituted phenethylamine family, sharing a core phenethylamine skeleton with a methylenedioxy ring substitution (Green et al., 2003). This ring-substituted structure is critical to its ability to enhance serotonin release (Iversen et al., 2008). The compound's molecular formula is C11_{11}11H15_{15}15NO2_22, and it is classified as a racemic mixture (R/S enantiomers) in many preparations. Both enantiomers can contribute differently to MDMA's overall psychoactive profile:

- **R(-)-MDMA** may exhibit slightly stronger empathogenic and entactogenic qualities.
- **S(+)-MDMA** can have a more pronounced stimulant effect (Ensslin et al., 2008).

While these enantiomeric variations can influence subjective experience, most clinical and illicit MDMA formulations contain both enantiomers in variable ratios (de la Torre et al., 2000).

## Monoamine Release and Reuptake Inhibition

MDMA's primary mechanism involves binding to monoamine transporters (e.g., SERT, DAT, NET) and reversing their function, causing an acute influx of serotonin, dopamine, and norepinephrine into the synaptic cleft (Green et al., 2003). This surge in monoamines correlates with elevated mood, increased sociability, and reduced fear responses:

1. **Serotonin (5-HT):** The substantial release of serotonin underpins much of MDMA's euphoria, heightened empathy, and prosocial behavior.
2. **Dopamine (DA):** Dopamine release contributes to mild stimulant effects, including elevated energy and, in some cases, a moderate risk for misuse or dependency (Schenk, 2011).
3. **Norepinephrine (NE):** Increased norepinephrine drives sympathomimetic responses, such as increased heart rate and blood pressure (Kirkpatrick et al., 2014).

Simultaneously, MDMA partially inhibits the reuptake mechanisms for these neurotransmitters, further prolonging their synaptic presence. The net result is a powerful, though relatively short-lived, increase in mood, emotional openness, and energy (Liechti & Vollenweider, 2001).

## Receptor Affinities and Secondary Targets

Beyond transporter-mediated release, MDMA exhibits lower-affinity interactions with various receptor subtypes, including 5-HT2_22 and α1_11 -adrenergic receptors (Green et al., 2003). While these effects are less pronounced than those of classical psychedelics at 5-HT2_22 sites, they can contribute to mild perceptual changes—such as enhanced color or texture perception—as well as to certain physiological side effects like vasoconstriction (Mueller et al., 2016).

## Pharmacokinetics

The onset of MDMA's effects typically begins within 30–45 minutes, peaking around 60–90 minutes, and gradually subsiding after 3–5 hours (de la Torre et al., 2000). Metabolic pathways predominantly involve the liver enzyme CYP2D6, which converts MDMA into various metabolites (Green et al., 2003). Genetic polymorphisms in CYP2D6 can influence the duration and intensity of MDMA's effects, making certain individuals more susceptible to adverse outcomes such as hyperthermia or prolonged cardiovascular strain (Van Dongen et al., 2020).

---

## References


- Carhart-Harris, R. L., & Goodwin, G. M. (2017). The therapeutic potential of psychedelic drugs: Past, present, and future. *Neuropsychopharmacology*, 42(11), 2105–2113.
- de la Torre, R., Farre, M., Roset, P. N., Pizarro, N., Abanades, S., Segura, M., ... Cami, J. (2000). Human pharmacology of MDMA: pharmacokinetics, metabolism, and disposition. *Therapeutic Drug Monitoring*, 22(1), 137–140.
- Ensslin, H. K., Kovar, K. A., Maurer, H. H. (2008). Metabolism of racemic MDMA and its enantiomers in humans: Systematic studies with authentic urine samples in comparison to rats and mice. *Therapeutic Drug Monitoring*, 30(4), 486–495.
- Green, A. R., Mechan, A. O., Elliott, J. M., O'Shea, E., & Colado, M. I. (2003). The pharmacology and clinical pharmacology of 3,4-

methylenedioxymethamphetamine (MDMA, "ecstasy"). *Pharmacological Reviews*, 55(3), 463–508.

- Iversen, L., Gibbons, S., Treble, R., Setola, V., Huang, X. P., & Roth, B. L. (2008). Neurochemical profiles of some novel psychoactive substances. *European Journal of Pharmacology*, 700(1–3), 147–151.
- Kirkpatrick, M. G., Gunderson, E. W., Perez, A. Y., Haney, M., Foltin, R. W., & Hart, C. L. (2014). A direct comparison of the behavioral and physiological effects of methamphetamine and 3,4-methylenedioxymethamphetamine (MDMA) in humans. *Psychopharmacology*, 231(22), 4241–4252.
- Liechti, M. E., & Vollenweider, F. X. (2001). Which neuroreceptors mediate the subjective effects of MDMA in humans? A summary of current knowledge. *Progress in Neuro-Psychopharmacology & Biological Psychiatry*, 25(4), 871–881.
- Mueller, F., Lenz, C., Dolder, P. C., Harder, S., Schmid, Y., Lang, U. E., & Liechti, M. E. (2016). Acute effects of MDMA and methylphenidate on error-related brain activity in healthy subjects. *Psychopharmacology*, 233(3), 355–363.
- Nichols, D. E. (1986). Differences between the mechanism of action of MDMA, MBDB, and the classic hallucinogens: Identification of a new therapeutic class. *Journal of Psychoactive Drugs*, 18(4), 305–313.
- Schenk, S. (2011). MDMA ("ecstasy") abuse as an example of dopamine neuroplasticity. *Neuroscience & Biobehavioral Reviews*, 35(5), 1203–1218.
- Van Dongen, M. C., Verkes, R. J., & Kahn, R. S. (2020). Does metabolism matter? The role of cytochrome P450 variation in MDMA-related drug effects and toxicity. *Drug Metabolism Reviews*, 52(2), 231–247.

# 3.2 Neurological and Psychological Effects of MDMA

In exploring MDMA's impact on the brain and on subjective experience, it is vital to examine both the immediate neurochemical changes and the broader psychological outcomes. Similar to discussions around psilocybin and LSD, MDMA's effects extend from measurable alterations in limbic structures (e.g., the amygdala) to significant shifts in emotional processing and interpersonal awareness (Gamma et al., 2000; Hysek et al., 2014). This chapter provides an overview of these changes, highlighting the acute neurological responses, the unique empathogenic qualities of MDMA, and the potential long-term psychological implications.

## Acute Neurological Effects

**Serotonin, Dopamine, and Norepinephrine Release**

MDMA's primary pharmacological action is the increased release and reuptake inhibition of serotonin, dopamine, and norepinephrine in the brain (Mithoefer et al., 2011). Elevated serotonin levels are most closely associated with mood enhancement and a sense of well-being. Dopamine adds stimulating properties, while norepinephrine contributes to heightened alertness and, in some cases, elevated heart rate and blood pressure.

**Amygdala Attenuation and Fear Response**

One of MDMA's most notable effects is its ability to modulate activity in the amygdala, an area of the brain closely linked with fear processing (Gamma et al., 2000). Under the influence of MDMA, amygdala hyperactivity in response to negative or threatening stimuli appears reduced, potentially allowing individuals—particularly those with trauma histories—to revisit painful memories without becoming overwhelmed (Mithoefer et al., 2011). By dampening the intensity of fear reactions, MDMA can foster a safer space for emotional exploration and therapeutic breakthroughs.

## Enhanced Emotional Processing and Empathy

**Prosocial and Empathogenic Qualities**

MDMA is often described as an "empathogen" due to its reliable enhancement of empathy, closeness, and prosocial behaviors (Bedi et al., 2010). Clinical and laboratory studies have consistently shown increased emotional sensitivity and improved recognition of both positive and negative emotional states in others (Hysek et al., 2014). These findings underscore MDMA's unique therapeutic value in psychotherapy settings, where emotional openness and trust are paramount.

**Subjective Emotional Warmth**

Alongside measurable prosocial shifts, many users report feelings of warmth, love, and compassion toward others—emotions that can be especially beneficial in therapeutic contexts for addressing interpersonal conflict or attachment-related trauma (Sessa, 2017). However, these effects are dose-dependent and can vary based on individual characteristics such as baseline emotional resilience, mental health status, and prior experiences.

## Increased Brain Connectivity and Cognitive Shifts

**Network Interactions**

Beyond its effects on the amygdala, MDMA appears to influence overall functional connectivity in the brain. Neuroimaging studies have shown altered connectivity between limbic regions and higher-order cortical areas, thereby facilitating emotional introspection and cognitive reframing (Gamma et al., 2000). By reducing the "filter" or "defensive" response to stressful memories, MDMA-assisted therapy can encourage patients to confront and integrate traumatic experiences more effectively (Mithoefer et al., 2011).

**Cognitive Bias and Reappraisal**

The heightened emotional state induced by MDMA may also reduce negative cognitive biases, enabling a more balanced self-assessment and empathy for others (Bedi et al., 2010). While some cognitive functions, such as working memory, may be slightly impaired during the acute phase, the overarching tendency is a shift toward prosocial cognition and positive affect, which can have profound therapeutic implications when guided by skilled professionals (Hysek et al., 2014).

## Potential Long-Term Implications and Risks

### Therapeutic Window for Emotional Healing

When used in controlled clinical environments, MDMA's empathogenic properties can create a therapeutic window for addressing deep-seated emotional wounds. Research indicates that MDMA-assisted psychotherapy may offer lasting relief for treatment-resistant conditions, particularly PTSD, by enabling patients to process traumatic memories without acute terror (Mithoefer et al., 2011; Sessa, 2021).

### Neurotoxicity and Safety Considerations

Despite MDMA's promising therapeutic profile, concerns about neurotoxicity have persisted. Studies suggest that toxic outcomes are more commonly linked to excessive or frequent recreational use, especially at high doses or in overheated, dehydrating conditions (Hysek et al., 2014). Under clinically monitored settings with appropriate dosage protocols and medical screening, the risk of neurotoxic damage appears substantially lower (Sessa, 2017). Nonetheless, ongoing research is required to fully understand MDMA's long-term safety profile, particularly for vulnerable populations and repeated therapeutic sessions.

## Conclusion

MDMA elicits a complex interplay of neurochemical, emotional, and cognitive effects that set it apart from classical psychedelics. Through increased serotonin and reduced amygdala reactivity, individuals may experience diminished fear, enhanced empathy, and stronger therapeutic rapport—a combination that can be transformative in addressing trauma, anxiety, and relational issues (Bedi et al., 2010; Sessa, 2017). While acute elevations in heart rate, body temperature, and mild cognitive impairments can occur, these changes generally remain manageable within clinical settings. As research continues, MDMA's ability to both soften emotional defenses and bolster interpersonal connection underscores its emerging role in modern psychiatry and trauma-focused therapy (Mithoefer et al., 2011; Hysek et al., 2014).

## References


- Bedi, G., Hyman, D., & De Wit, H. (2010). Is ecstasy an "empathogen"? Effects of ±3,4-methylenedioxymethamphetamine on prosocial feelings and identification of emotional states in others. *Biological Psychiatry, 68*(12), 1134–1140.
- Gamma, A., Buck, A., Berthold, T., Liechti, M. E., & Vollenweider, F. X. (2000). 3,4-Methylenedioxymethamphetamine (MDMA) modulates cortical and limbic activation measured by positron emission tomography (PET) in healthy humans. *Neuropsychopharmacology, 23*(4), 388–395.
- Hysek, C. M., Schmid, Y., Simmler, L. D., Domes, G., Heinrichs, M., Eisenegger, C., ... Liechti, M. E. (2014). MDMA enhances emotional empathy and prosocial behavior. *Social Cognitive and Affective Neuroscience, 9*(11), 1645–1652.
- Mithoefer, M. C., Wagner, M. T., Mithoefer, A. T., Jerome, I., & Doblin, R. (2011). The safety and efficacy of ±3,4-methylenedioxymethamphetamine-assisted psychotherapy in subjects with chronic, treatment-resistant posttraumatic stress disorder: The first randomized controlled pilot study. *Journal of Psychopharmacology, 25*(4), 439–452.
- Sessa, B. (2017). MDMA and PTSD treatment: 'PTSD: From novel pathophysiology to innovative therapeutics'. *Journal of Psychopharmacology, 31*(10), 1101–1111.
- Sessa, B. (2021). The 21st-century psychedelic renaissance: Heroic steps forward on the back of an elephant. *Psychopharmacology, 238*(1), 29–42.

## 3.3 Physical and Psychological Effects of MDMA

In examining MDMA's profile, it is essential to address the full spectrum of its effects on both the body and mind. While much attention has focused on MDMA's potential as a therapeutic agent for conditions such as PTSD, understanding its acute physiological responses and the depth of its psychological impact is equally important. This chapter explores the common physical changes that occur during MDMA use, the broad range of subjective experiences, and the longer-term psychological outcomes reported in clinical and non-clinical settings (Mithoefer et al., 2011; Hysek et al., 2014).

### Acute Physical Effects

#### Vital Signs and Autonomic Responses

Similar to other psychoactive substances, MDMA can produce noticeable changes in vital signs. Users often experience elevated heart rate, increases in blood pressure, and mild shifts in body temperature, reflecting its sympathomimetic activity (Liechti, 2014). These physiological responses are generally transient and may be more pronounced at higher doses or in warm, crowded conditions such as dance venues (Bedi et al., 2010). From a clinical standpoint, understanding these autonomic changes is critical, especially for individuals with pre-existing cardiovascular concerns (Mithoefer et al., 2011). Monitoring and appropriate medical screening can help mitigate risks in therapeutic settings.

#### Sensory and Somatic Perceptions

MDMA also influences the sensory experience, often amplifying tactile sensations and producing a heightened sense of bodily awareness (Hysek et al., 2014). Some individuals describe a warming or tingling sensation throughout the body, accompanied by changes in muscle tension or jaw clenching. In rare cases or at higher doses, nausea or mild gastrointestinal discomfort can occur, though these effects typically subside as the acute phase ends (Kuypers et al., 2017).

## Acute Psychological Effects

### Emotional Euphoria and Empathy

Unlike classical psychedelics such as psilocybin or LSD, MDMA is categorized as an entactogen or empathogen, primarily due to its marked enhancement of emotional warmth and empathetic understanding (Bedi et al., 2010). Clinically, these effects are especially relevant when assisting patients in exploring traumatic experiences, as the reduction in fear responses can facilitate more open communication (Mithoefer et al., 2011). Many users report profound feelings of closeness and connectedness, which, in therapeutic contexts, can foster a safe environment for emotional release (Hysek et al., 2014).

### Potential for Anxiety or Dysphoria

Although MDMA is often associated with positive mood elevation, instances of anxiety, restlessness, or transient dysphoria can occur (Kuypers et al., 2017). These adverse effects may be precipitated by high doses, dehydration, or suboptimal set and setting, emphasizing the importance of careful dose management and supportive supervision (Sessa, 2017). In a controlled therapeutic framework, such moments of discomfort can be navigated proactively, transforming challenging episodes into therapeutic opportunities.

## Longer-Term Psychological Effects

### Therapeutic Aftermath

Beyond the immediate experience, MDMA's empathogenic qualities can yield notable post-session reflections, often described as increased self-compassion, reduced avoidance of difficult memories, and an expanded sense of emotional openness (Mithoefer et al., 2011). In clinical trials, these aftereffects have been linked with sustained improvements in PTSD symptoms and overall psychological well-being, particularly when supported by integrative psychotherapy sessions (Schmid & Liechti, 2018).

### Neurocognitive Considerations

While concerns about MDMA-related neurotoxicity have circulated in popular media, research suggests that long-term neurocognitive deficits are more commonly associated with high-dose recreational use rather than controlled clinical administration (Sessa, 2017). Studies tracking cognitive performance over time generally indicate minimal lasting impairment when MDMA is employed in therapeutic doses, alongside thorough screening and harm-reduction strategies (Kuypers et al., 2017).

**Risks and Potential for Misuse**

Even in medical contexts, it is crucial to acknowledge the potential for misuse. Repeated or excessive use of MDMA—particularly in unregulated settings—may contribute to mood disturbances, including "midweek blues" or a temporary "comedown" effect marked by low mood and fatigue (Bedi et al., 2010). These risks underscore the need for clear guidelines, rigorous patient selection, and structured follow-up when integrating MDMA into psychotherapeutic protocols (Mithoefer et al., 2011).

## Conclusion

MDMA exerts a distinctive range of physical and psychological effects, from transient autonomic changes to profound experiences of empathy and emotional relief. In clinical environments, these properties can catalyze significant therapeutic breakthroughs, particularly in trauma-related disorders. Nonetheless, vigilance around cardiovascular health, psychological preparedness, and potential for misuse remains essential. As evidence-based research continues to evolve, MDMA's empathogenic and fear-reducing effects position it as a promising agent in modern psychiatry—provided it is administered responsibly and under professional oversight (Sessa, 2017; Schmid & Liechti, 2018).

## References


- Bedi, G., Hyman, D., & de Wit, H. (2010). Is ecstasy an "empathogen"? Effects of ±3,4-methylenedioxymethamphetamine on prosocial feelings and identification of emotional states in others. *Biological Psychiatry, 68*(12), 1134–1140.
- Hysek, C. M., Schmid, Y., Simmler, L. D., Domes, G., Heinrichs, M., et al. (2014). MDMA enhances "emotional empathy" and prosocial behavior. *Social Cognitive and Affective Neuroscience, 9*(11), 1645–1652.

- Kuypers, K. P. C., De La Torre, R., Farre, M., Pujadas, M., Navines, R., et al. (2017). Inhibition of MDMA-induced increase in cortisol does not prevent negative effects on cognitive performance. *Pharmacopsychiatry, 50*(1), 17–23.
- Liechti, M. E. (2014). Effects of MDMA on body temperature in humans. *Temperature, 1*(3), 191–193.
- Mithoefer, M. C., Wagner, M. T., Mithoefer, A. T., Jerome, I., & Doblin, R. (2011). The safety and efficacy of ±3,4-methylenedioxymethamphetamine-assisted psychotherapy in subjects with chronic, treatment-resistant posttraumatic stress disorder: The first randomized controlled pilot study. *Journal of Psychopharmacology, 25*(4), 439–452.
- Schmid, Y., & Liechti, M. E. (2018). Long-lasting subjective effects of a single dose of MDMA and 14 months follow-up. *Journal of Psychopharmacology, 32*(11), 1198–1205.
- Sessa, B. (2017). MDMA and PTSD treatment: 'PTSD: from novel pathophysiology to innovative therapeutics.' *Neuropharmacology, 142,* 254–260.

# Chapter 4. Clinical Research and Therapeutic Potential of MDMA

MDMA (±3,4-methylenedioxymethamphetamine) has garnered significant attention within the psychiatric community due to its potential to facilitate therapeutic breakthroughs, particularly for individuals with treatment-resistant conditions. Over the past four decades, early anecdotal reports have gradually transformed into rigorous clinical investigations, culminating in the current wave of FDA-approved clinical trials for posttraumatic stress disorder (PTSD) and other mental health conditions (Mithoefer et al., 2011; Jerome et al., 2020). This chapter explores the evolution of MDMA research—from its initial therapeutic use in the late 1970s to modern, large-scale clinical trials—and examines how these findings inform the broader therapeutic potential of MDMA.

## Early Therapeutic Observations

Before MDMA became synonymous with "ecstasy" in the 1980s, its therapeutic potential was noted by psychotherapists who observed that it promoted emotional openness and reduced fear-based responses (Greer & Tolbert, 1986). Although these early applications were largely informal and lacked systematic data collection, anecdotal successes—especially in treating trauma and anxiety—prompted further interest among clinicians and researchers (Sessa, 2017).

## Emergence of Rigorous Clinical Protocols

Following the prohibition of MDMA in 1985, scientific investigations stalled, and knowledge of MDMA's clinical benefits shifted to underground therapy circles (Doblin, 2002). However, through persistent advocacy, organizations like the Multidisciplinary Association for Psychedelic Studies (MAPS) launched a series of pilot studies in the early 2000s (Mithoefer et al., 2011). These studies adhered to strict clinical protocols, including:

- **Screening and Preparation:** Participants underwent medical evaluations to rule out contraindications (e.g., severe cardiac conditions).

- **MDMA-Assisted Sessions:** Therapeutic sessions incorporated moderate doses of MDMA (typically 75–125 mg), administered in a controlled clinical environment with trained therapists.
- **Integration Phases:** Follow-up sessions focused on helping participants process and integrate emotional insights gained during the MDMA experience.

Collectively, these pilot studies demonstrated both the safety and preliminary efficacy of MDMA-assisted psychotherapy, particularly for individuals with chronic, treatment-resistant PTSD (Mithoefer et al., 2011; Oehen et al., 2013).

## FDA Breakthrough Therapy Status

In 2017, the U.S. Food and Drug Administration (FDA) granted MDMA-assisted psychotherapy a "Breakthrough Therapy" designation, expediting research efforts for PTSD (Multidisciplinary Association for Psychedelic Studies [MAPS], 2021). This status acknowledges MDMA's potential to offer substantial advantages over existing treatments and paves the way for larger Phase 3 trials. These pivotal trials aim to establish efficacy and safety in more diverse populations and clinical settings, incorporating robust methodologies such as randomized controlled designs and stringent data monitoring protocols (Jerome et al., 2020).

## Efficacy Across Diagnostic Categories

Although much of the current research focuses on PTSD, emerging data suggest that MDMA-assisted therapy may benefit conditions marked by deep-seated emotional dysregulation or relational conflicts:

- **Depression and Anxiety:** Preliminary case reports and ongoing trials indicate that MDMA's empathogenic qualities could alleviate symptoms of major depressive disorder and social anxiety (Amoroso & Workman, 2016).

- **Addiction:** Exploratory studies propose that MDMA's facilitation of emotional openness may help address underlying trauma or relational stressors contributing to substance use disorders (Sessa, 2017).
- **Couples Therapy:** Early anecdotal evidence points to MDMA's capacity for enhancing empathy and communication between partners, prompting interest in structured, therapist-led interventions for relational distress (Wagner et al., 2021).

### Remaining Challenges and Future Directions

Despite promising findings, several challenges remain:

- **Safety and Contraindications:** MDMA may pose risks for individuals with cardiovascular issues, bipolar disorder, or psychotic-spectrum disorders. Thorough screening is therefore essential (Jerome et al., 2020).
- **Therapist Training and Accessibility:** As MDMA approaches potential legalization for clinical use, standardized training programs will be needed to ensure ethical and effective administration (MAPS, 2021).
- **Long-Term Efficacy:** Sustained benefits require robust integration frameworks and follow-up protocols to consolidate therapeutic insights gained under MDMA (Mithoefer et al., 2019).

Collectively, these concerns reflect the need for further research and regulatory adaptations. Nonetheless, MDMA has demonstrated a remarkable capacity for facilitating emotional breakthroughs, particularly in populations unresponsive to traditional therapies.

## 4.1 Early and Modern Research on MDMA-Assisted Therapy

In order to appreciate the current landscape of MDMA research, it is instructive to examine the developmental trajectory of investigations—from informal, pre-prohibition explorations to the structured clinical trials of the present day. This section delves deeper into the foundational studies, the evolution of protocols, and the clinical findings that have shaped modern MDMA-assisted therapy.

## Pre-Prohibition Studies and Informal Applications

During the late 1970s and early 1980s, psychotherapists like Leo Zeff and others administered MDMA (often referred to as "Adam") within therapeutic contexts to foster emotional connectivity and decrease anxiety (Greer & Tolbert, 1986). Though methodologically limited, these informal trials provided a framework for understanding how MDMA might enhance empathy and trust, particularly in trauma-focused therapy (Doblin, 2002).

## Post-Prohibition Pilot Studies

Once MDMA was classified as a Schedule I substance in the United States (1985), sanctioned research stopped for nearly two decades (Doblin, 2002). It was not until the late 1990s and early 2000s that MAPS and other research bodies received approvals to conduct small-scale, pilot trials.

- **Design and Outcomes:** Pioneering studies employed a randomized, double-blind, placebo-controlled model to examine MDMA's safety and efficacy in individuals diagnosed with chronic PTSD (Mithoefer et al., 2011). Results indicated statistically significant reductions in PTSD symptom severity, maintained during long-term follow-up (Mithoefer et al., 2019).
- **Psychotherapeutic Process:** Researchers noted that MDMA facilitated engagement with traumatic memories by reducing fear response and amplifying emotional processing, thus allowing patients to revisit traumatic events without becoming overwhelmed (Amoroso & Workman, 2016).

## Modern Clinical Trials and Multicenter Collaborations

Building on the success of pilot studies, large-scale Phase 2 and Phase 3 trials have been conducted across multiple centers in the United States, Canada,

Israel, and Europe (Jerome et al., 2020). These trials incorporate rigorous screening protocols, standardized dosing regimens, and manualized therapy sessions to ensure reproducibility.

- **Global Research Networks:** Collaborations among researchers, non-profit organizations, and academic institutions have accelerated data sharing and contributed to a standardized approach in administering MDMA-assisted psychotherapy.
- **Preliminary Meta-Analyses:** Although meta-analytical data on MDMA are still limited compared to some established pharmacotherapies, emerging reviews point toward a consistently positive effect on PTSD symptoms (Sessa, 2017).

## Implications for Broader Psychiatric Practice

The trajectory of MDMA research exemplifies how a once-stigmatized compound can transition into a legitimate psychotherapeutic agent when supported by systematic investigations and compelling clinical data. As larger trials conclude and regulatory bodies evaluate the results, MDMA stands on the cusp of being fully integrated into mainstream psychiatric practice—offering new avenues for treating trauma and potentially other mental health conditions (Jerome et al., 2020).

---

## References


- Amoroso, T., & Workman, M. (2016). Treating posttraumatic stress disorder with MDMA-assisted psychotherapy: A preliminary meta-analysis and comparison to prolonged exposure therapy. *Journal of Psychopharmacology*, 30(7), 595–600.
- Doblin, R. (2002). A clinical plan for MDMA (ecstasy) in the treatment of posttraumatic stress disorder (PTSD): Partnering with the FDA. *Journal of Psychoactive Drugs*, 34(2), 185–194.
- Greer, G., & Tolbert, R. (1986). Subjective reports of the effects of MDMA in a clinical setting. *Journal of Psychoactive Drugs*, 18(4), 319–327.

- Jerome, I., Feduccia, A. A., & Mithoefer, M. C. (2020). MDMA-assisted psychotherapy for the treatment of posttraumatic stress disorder: Findings from recent trials and implications for clinical practice. *Current Psychiatry Reports*, 22(5), 25–34.
- MAPS (Multidisciplinary Association for Psychedelic Studies). (2021). *MDMA Research Timeline*. Retrieved from https://maps.org
- Mithoefer, M. C., Wagner, M. T., Mithoefer, A. T., Jerome, I., & Doblin, R. (2011). The safety and efficacy of ±3,4-methylenedioxymethamphetamine-assisted psychotherapy in subjects with chronic, treatment-resistant posttraumatic stress disorder: The first randomized controlled pilot study. *Journal of Psychopharmacology*, 25(4), 439–452.
- Mithoefer, M. C., Jerome, I., & Doblin, R. (2019). MDMA-assisted psychotherapy for treatment of PTSD: A model for future research and drug development. *Frontiers in Psychiatry*, 10, 650–662.
- Oehen, P., Traber, R., Widmer, V., & Schnyder, U. (2013). A pilot study on ±3,4-methylenedioxymethamphetamine (MDMA)-assisted psychotherapy for anxiety associated with life-threatening illnesses. *Journal of Psychopharmacology*, 27(5), 442–450.
- Sessa, B. (2017). MDMA and PTSD treatment: "PTSD: From novel pathophysiology to innovative therapeutics." *Neuropharmacology*, 142, 254–260.
- Wagner, A. C., Lau, T., & Schulz-Heik, R. (2021). Couples therapy and MDMA: A scoping review of the theory and potential applications. *Journal of Psychoactive Drugs*, 53(2), 115–125.

## 4.2 MDMA for PTSD and Trauma Processing

In examining MDMA's therapeutic role in addressing post-traumatic stress disorder (PTSD), it is crucial to explore both the neurobiological underpinnings that make it uniquely effective and the structured clinical approaches that have demonstrated promising outcomes. This chapter delves into how MDMA appears to reduce hypervigilance, foster emotional safety, and facilitate the reprocessing of traumatic memories—elements that have positioned MDMA-assisted psychotherapy as a potential breakthrough in trauma care (Mithoefer et al., 2011; Sessa, 2017).

### Mechanisms of Fear Extinction

A defining characteristic of PTSD is the persistent reactivity to trauma-related cues, often manifesting as flashbacks, nightmares, and hyperarousal (Bisson et al., 2021). MDMA's acute pharmacological effects—chiefly its ability to increase serotonin, dopamine, and norepinephrine—contribute to a state of emotional openness that can interrupt entrenched fear responses (Jerome et al., 2020). Neuroimaging studies suggest that MDMA modulates activity in the amygdala, diminishing fear-related processing while enhancing connectivity in brain regions associated with emotional regulation and memory integration (Carhart-Harris et al., 2015; Mithoefer et al., 2018). These neurobiological shifts help patients engage with traumatic material more directly, reducing avoidance behaviors and supporting a reclassification of painful memories.

### Therapeutic Efficacy and Emotional Safety

In contrast to classic psychedelics such as psilocybin or LSD—which often induce visionary or hallucinatory states—MDMA produces empathogenic and prosocial effects, including heightened trust and reduced defensiveness (Sessa, 2017). By attenuating fear and increasing feelings of emotional safety, MDMA allows patients to revisit traumatic memories without becoming overwhelmed (Feduccia & Mithoefer, 2018). This emotional buffer encourages deeper therapeutic engagement, where the patient can explore, process, and ultimately reframe traumatic experiences within a structured setting (Mithoefer et al.,

2011). Notably, this process does not eliminate negative emotions entirely; rather, it provides a manageable context in which these emotions can be acknowledged, understood, and integrated.

## Clinical Protocols: Preparation, Dosing, and Integration

Similar to psilocybin-assisted therapies, the MDMA treatment model typically encompasses three core phases: preparation, the MDMA-assisted session(s), and post-session integration (Mithoefer et al., 2018).

1. **Preparation**
   Patients undergo thorough medical and psychological screenings to rule out contraindications such as severe cardiovascular disorders or psychotic spectrum conditions. A stable and trusting therapeutic relationship is established, and the patient is briefed on what to expect from MDMA's psychoactive effects (Jerome et al., 2020).
2. **MDMA-Assisted Session**
   On the day of the session, patients generally receive a dose ranging from 75 to 125 mg of pharmaceutical-grade MDMA, followed by optional supplemental dosing after a set period to prolong therapeutic windows (Mithoefer et al., 2018). During the 6–8-hour session, trained therapists provide emotional support, encourage exploration of difficult memories, and employ psychotherapeutic techniques such as internal focus, somatic awareness, or guided imagery. Unlike psilocybin-induced visions, MDMA prompts introspective clarity while preserving a relatively clear sensorium—an attribute that helps patients articulate their emotional experiences in real time (Sessa, 2017).
3. **Integration**
   Following the session, one or more integration appointments help patients process insights, address unresolved emotional content, and develop coping strategies for daily life (Feduccia & Mithoefer, 2018). This phase is critical, as it bridges the gap between the acute experience and long-term psychological change (Jerome et al., 2020).

## Challenges and Considerations

While MDMA-assisted psychotherapy for PTSD has gained momentum, it is not without risks or limitations. Concerns include transient increases in heart rate and blood pressure, potential for emotional overload if underlying trauma is especially severe, and the necessity of highly trained therapists to manage acute distress or difficult memories (Mithoefer et al., 2018; Sessa, 2017). Moreover, the illegality of MDMA in many jurisdictions currently restricts widespread clinical implementation. Rigorous protocols, therapist training programs, and risk mitigation measures remain central to ethical and effective practice (Feduccia & Mithoefer, 2018).

## Conclusion

MDMA's unique empathogenic profile offers a promising therapeutic avenue for individuals grappling with PTSD, where emotional numbing and fear responses often hinder healing. By fostering an environment conducive to introspection and emotional safety, MDMA-assisted psychotherapy has the potential to catalyze meaningful shifts in how patients process and integrate traumatic memories. As ongoing research continues to validate both the efficacy and safety of this approach, MDMA stands on the brink of transforming the landscape of trauma treatment—underscoring the importance of further clinical trials, policy reform, and professional education (Mithoefer et al., 2018; Jerome et al., 2020).

## References


- Bisson, J. I., Cosgrove, S., Lewis, C., & Roberts, N. P. (2021). Post-traumatic stress disorder. *BMJ*, 372, n94.
- Carhart-Harris, R. L., Wall, M. B., et al. (2015). The effects of acute MDMA on brain responses to fearful faces in humans. *Social Cognitive and Affective Neuroscience*, 10(12), 1697–1705.
- Feduccia, A. A., & Mithoefer, M. C. (2018). MDMA-assisted psychotherapy for PTSD: Are memory reconsolidation and fear extinction underlying mechanisms? *Progress in Neuro-Psychopharmacology & Biological Psychiatry*, 84(Pt A), 221–228.

- Jerome, I., Yazar-Klosinski, B., et al. (2020). Long-term follow-up outcomes of MDMA-assisted psychotherapy for treatment of PTSD: A longitudinal pooled analysis of six phase 2 trials. *Psychopharmacology*, 237(8), 2485–2497.
- Mithoefer, M. C., Wagner, M. T., Mithoefer, A. T., Jerome, I., & Doblin, R. (2011). The safety and efficacy of ±3,4-methylenedioxymethamphetamine-assisted psychotherapy in subjects with chronic, treatment-resistant posttraumatic stress disorder: The first randomized controlled pilot study. *Journal of Psychopharmacology*, 25(4), 439–452.
- Mithoefer, M. C., Mithoefer, A. T., Feduccia, A. A., Jerome, I., Wagner, M. T., Wymer, J., ... Doblin, R. (2018). 3,4-Methylenedioxymethamphetamine (MDMA)-assisted psychotherapy for post-traumatic stress disorder in military veterans, firefighters, and police officers: A randomized, double-blind, dose-response, Phase 2 clinical trial. *Lancet Psychiatry*, 5(6), 486–497.
- Sessa, B. (2017). MDMA and PTSD treatment: "PTSD: From novel pathophysiology to innovative therapeutics." *Neurotherapeutics*, 14(3), 612–622.

# 4.3 Comparing MDMA to Other Therapeutic Agents

In evaluating MDMA's therapeutic potential, it is critical to situate it within the broader landscape of psychiatric treatments. While selective serotonin reuptake inhibitors (SSRIs) have long been considered a mainstay for managing mood and anxiety disorders (Cipriani et al., 2018), and classical psychedelics like psilocybin and LSD are gaining renewed attention for their transformative effects on cognition and self-perception (Carhart-Harris et al., 2018), MDMA occupies a unique niche. This section examines how MDMA contrasts with these established treatments in terms of pharmacological mechanisms, therapeutic outcomes, and clinical considerations (Mithoefer et al., 2019; Sessa, 2017).

## MDMA vs. SSRIs

**Mechanistic Differences**

SSRIs alleviate symptoms of depression and anxiety primarily by increasing extracellular serotonin levels through reuptake inhibition, leading to gradual mood stabilization (Cipriani et al., 2018). However, they often dampen emotional range and can be accompanied by side effects such as sexual dysfunction, weight gain, and emotional blunting (Fava, 2018). MDMA, on the other hand, acutely increases the release of serotonin, dopamine, and norepinephrine—resulting in a more immediate enhancement of empathy, sociability, and emotional openness (de la Torre et al., 2004).

**Therapeutic Implications**

By amplifying emotional experiences rather than modulating them over time, MDMA-assisted therapy can facilitate profound introspective and interpersonal breakthroughs in a comparatively short number of sessions (Mithoefer et al., 2019). This heightened emotional clarity is particularly valuable for processing trauma, as patients can revisit painful experiences without the intense fear response that typically accompanies them (Jerome et al., 2020). However, the intensity of MDMA's effects also underscores the need for careful medical screening, a controlled environment, and thorough integration support, whereas SSRIs can be administered more widely in outpatient contexts with less acute monitoring (Bedi et al., 2009).

## MDMA vs. Classical Psychedelics

### Phenomenological Profile

Classical psychedelics such as psilocybin and LSD predominantly act on the 5-HT2A receptor, often inducing perceptual distortions, visionary experiences, and the possibility of ego dissolution (Carhart-Harris & Goodwin, 2017). MDMA, while it also influences serotonin pathways, is not generally classified as a classic psychedelic because it does not reliably produce vivid hallucinations or profound disruptions of visual perception (Nichols, 2016). Instead, it is best described as an "empathogen" or "entactogen," enhancing pro-social emotions, empathy, and self-acceptance (Sessa, 2017).

### Clinical Considerations

The reduced likelihood of intense perceptual shifts makes MDMA potentially more predictable for certain populations, including individuals who might be hesitant to engage with the radical perceptual changes associated with classical psychedelics (Nutt & Carhart-Harris, 2021). However, some therapeutic frameworks specifically value the "mystical" or "transcendent" components of psilocybin and LSD sessions for catalyzing deep psychological insights (Johnson & Griffiths, 2017). In contrast, MDMA's more consistent emotional-opening profile may be particularly apt for structured trauma work, couples therapy, and social anxiety interventions (Sessa, 2017).

## Clinical Synergies and Future Directions

### Potential for Combined or Sequential Therapies

There is growing interest in how MDMA and classical psychedelics might complement each other in therapeutic settings—although empirical data remain limited (Nutt & Carhart-Harris, 2021). For instance, MDMA's emphasis on emotional bonding and catharsis could prepare patients for the more abstract or existential explorations often triggered by psilocybin or LSD sessions. Conversely, a prior psilocybin experience might facilitate deeper emotional processing during an MDMA session, as a patient may already have developed trust in non-ordinary states of consciousness (Carhart-Harris et al., 2018).

**Evolving Therapeutic Landscape**

As expanded access protocols become more established, the psychiatric community may begin to see a diversification of psychedelic-assisted therapies, each targeting different aspects of mental health (Carhart-Harris & Goodwin, 2017). MDMA's unique ability to foster emotional safety and interpersonal connectedness may be particularly relevant for disorders rooted in trauma and relational distress. Continued research comparing MDMA with SSRIs, classical psychedelics, and other novel agents will help clinicians make evidence-based decisions about personalized treatment pathways (Jerome et al., 2020; Mithoefer et al., 2019).

## Conclusion

MDMA's distinctive empathogenic qualities set it apart from both SSRIs and classical psychedelics, offering a promising avenue for rapid and deeply relational therapeutic interventions. Where SSRIs provide steady, long-term symptom management through neurochemical stabilization, MDMA delivers acute emotional openness that can accelerate trauma processing and interpersonal healing. Meanwhile, classical psychedelics offer opportunities for significant perceptual and existential insights, which may be less predictable but potentially transformative. As the field of psychedelic medicine continues to evolve, clarifying these comparative strengths and limitations will be essential for tailoring therapies to individual patient needs (Nutt & Carhart-Harris, 2021; Sessa, 2017).

## References


- Bedi, G., Van Dam, N. T., & Redman, J. (2009). Ecstasy (MDMA) and high trait empathy: Evidence for prosocial effects. Journal of Psychopharmacology, 23(4), 392–400.
- Carhart-Harris, R. L., Bolstridge, M., Day, C. M. J., et al. (2018). Psilocybin with psychological support for treatment-resistant depression: Six-month follow-up. Psychopharmacology, 235(2),

399–408.

- Carhart-Harris, R. L., & Goodwin, G. M. (2017). The therapeutic potential of psychedelic drugs: Past, present, and future. Neuropsychopharmacology, 42(11), 2105–2113.
- Cipriani, A., Furukawa, T. A., Salanti, G., et al. (2018). Comparative efficacy and acceptability of 21 antidepressant drugs for the acute treatment of adults with major depressive disorder: A systematic review and network meta-analysis. The Lancet, 391(10128), 1357–1366.
- de la Torre, R., Farré, M., Roset, P. N., et al. (2004). Human pharmacology of MDMA: Pharmacokinetics, metabolism, and disposition. Therapeutic Drug Monitoring, 26(2), 137–144.
- Fava, M. (2018). Weight gain and sexual dysfunction associated with SSRIs. Journal of Clinical Psychiatry, 79(2), 15–19.
- Jerome, I., Mithoefer, M. C., Feduccia, A. A., & Doblin, R. (2020). MDMA-assisted psychotherapy for the treatment of posttraumatic stress disorder: A review of current research and perspectives. Substance Abuse Rehabilitation, 11, 9–16.
- Johnson, M. W., & Griffiths, R. R. (2017). Potential therapeutic effects of psilocybin. Neurotherapeutics, 14(3), 734–740.
- Mithoefer, M. C., Mithoefer, A. T., Feduccia, A. A., et al. (2019). 3,4-Methylenedioxymethamphetamine (MDMA)-assisted psychotherapy for post-traumatic stress disorder in military veterans, firefighters, and police officers: A randomized, double-blind, dose-response, phase 2 clinical trial. The Lancet Psychiatry, 6(6), 475–485.
- Nichols, D. E. (2016). Psychedelics. Pharmacological Reviews, 68(2), 264–355.
- Nutt, D. J., & Carhart-Harris, R. (2021). The current status of psychedelics in psychiatry. JAMA Psychiatry, 78(2), 121–122.
- Sessa, B. (2017). MDMA therapy for PTSD and beyond. The Psychologist, 30, 42–47.

# Chapter 5. Therapeutic Applications for Psychiatrists

MDMA's emerging role in modern psychiatry is grounded in its capacity to facilitate emotional openness, reduce fear-based responses, and foster interpersonal connectedness (Mithoefer et al., 2011; Jerome et al., 2020). As growing research underscores MDMA's therapeutic benefits—particularly in posttraumatic stress disorder (PTSD)—psychiatrists are increasingly integrating MDMA into clinical paradigms. Yet, its application requires thorough patient evaluation, structured protocols, and a keen awareness of both medical and ethical considerations (Doblin et al., 2019; Sessa, 2017). This chapter provides an overview of MDMA-assisted therapy's scope, focusing on patient selection, common indications, and the safety measures essential for effective practice.

## 5.1 Indications and Patient Selection

In any therapeutic model, matching the treatment to the patient's needs is critical. The same holds true for MDMA-assisted therapy, where appropriate indication and rigorous screening can maximize benefits while minimizing potential harms (Feduccia & Mithoefer, 2018; Mithoefer et al., 2019). This section details the spectrum of psychiatric conditions where MDMA shows promise, along with contraindications and tools for patient assessment.

### Potential Psychiatric Indications

The bulk of MDMA's clinical evidence has concentrated on PTSD, but newer studies suggest applicability to a wider range of psychiatric issues (Jerome et al., 2020). Below are the key domains where MDMA-assisted therapy may offer therapeutic value.

**PTSD and Trauma-Related Disorders**

MDMA's best-supported indication lies in the treatment of PTSD (Mithoefer et al., 2011). By dampening the amygdala-driven fear response and enhancing empathetic connection, MDMA can enable patients to process traumatic memories with reduced emotional distress (Feduccia & Mithoefer, 2018). This mechanism has proven especially useful for individuals with chronic, treatment-resistant PTSD, yielding significant, and often enduring, symptom relief (Doblin et al., 2019).

**Depression and Anxiety Spectrum Disorders**

Beyond trauma-focused care, MDMA shows potential benefits in addressing major depressive disorder and generalized anxiety (Sessa, 2017). Some preliminary findings suggest that enhanced emotional insight, combined with a supportive therapeutic setting, may yield lasting improvements in mood and anxiety resilience (Jerome et al., 2020). Nonetheless, these results remain preliminary, highlighting the need for larger-scale controlled trials (Mithoefer et al., 2019).

**Social Anxiety and Relational Difficulties**

MDMA's empathogenic effects—elevated trust, decreased interpersonal defensiveness, and heightened emotional empathy—offer unique advantages for individuals struggling with social phobias or relational conflicts (Kuypers et al., 2017). In couples therapy, for example, MDMA has been noted to reduce communication barriers and foster mutual understanding, potentially accelerating relational healing (Wagner et al., 2019).

**End-of-Life Distress**

Similar to classical psychedelics, MDMA is under exploration for easing end-of-life anxiety in patients facing terminal illnesses (Sessa, 2017). While data are limited, early case reports indicate that the heightened sense of emotional safety and reduced existential fear can improve patients' psychological well-being, suggesting an important avenue for palliative care (Mithoefer et al., 2019).

## Contraindications and Cautionary Profiles

Despite MDMA's potential, not all patients stand to benefit. Certain medical and psychiatric conditions may raise the risk of severe adverse events, mandating a careful screening process (Vizeli & Liechti, 2017).

**Cardiovascular and Neurological Risks**

MDMA's stimulant properties can increase blood pressure, heart rate, and body temperature, posing concerns for individuals with cardiovascular or cerebrovascular disease (Sessa, 2017). Conditions like uncontrolled hypertension or a history of stroke typically contraindicate MDMA-assisted sessions (Doblin et al., 2019). Seizure disorders also warrant heightened caution or exclusion (Vizeli & Liechti, 2017).

**Severe Psychiatric Instability**

While MDMA may help manage trauma and mild-to-moderate anxiety or depression, patients with active psychosis, bipolar mania, or certain personality disorders should undergo comprehensive psychiatric evaluation before consideration (Carhart-Harris & Goodwin, 2017). For individuals with significant instability, alternative treatments—pharmacological or otherwise—should precede MDMA-assisted therapy (Sessa, 2017).

**Medication Interactions**

Because MDMA heavily influences serotonin release, concurrent use of monoamine oxidase inhibitors (MAOIs) or certain selective serotonin reuptake inhibitors (SSRIs) can heighten the risk of serotonin syndrome (Vizeli & Liechti, 2017). Psychiatrists must meticulously assess all prescribed and over-the-counter medications, including herbal supplements, that patients may be taking (Kuypers et al., 2017).

## Assessment and Screening Tools

A thorough intake process ensures patients are both medically and psychologically prepared for MDMA-assisted sessions (Mithoefer et al., 2019).

**Clinical Interviews and Psychometric Measures**

Structured interviews such as the Structured Clinical Interview for DSM-5 (SCID) can clarify diagnostic status and comorbidities (Doblin et al., 2019). Psychometric scales—covering PTSD severity, mood symptoms, or substance use—can further guide treatment planning and track outcome measures (Jerome et al., 2020).

**Medical Evaluations**

Baseline physical exams, including EKG and blood pressure monitoring, are essential to screen out potential cardiovascular vulnerabilities (Vizeli & Liechti, 2017). Laboratory tests—like liver function panels or electrolyte checks—can reveal issues that might compromise patient safety during MDMA sessions (Sessa, 2017).

**Informed Consent and Psychoeducation**

Central to ethical MDMA therapy is comprehensive patient education. Clinicians must clearly articulate the drug's effects, the structure of each session, and the importance of integration support (Mithoefer et al., 2011). This step ensures patients appreciate both the potential benefits and inherent uncertainties in MDMA-assisted therapy (Feduccia & Mithoefer, 2018).

## References


- Barrett, F. S., Johnson, M. W., & Griffiths, R. R. (2015). Validation of the revised Mystical Experience Questionnaire in experimental sessions with psilocybin. *Journal of Psychopharmacology, 29*(11), 1182–1190.
- Carhart-Harris, R. L., & Goodwin, G. M. (2017). The therapeutic potential of psychedelic drugs: Past, present, and future. *Neuropsychopharmacology, 42*(11), 2105–2113.
- Doblin, R., Christiansen, M., Jerome, I., & Burge, B. (2019). The past and future of MDMA-assisted psychotherapy for PTSD. *Journal of Psychopharmacology, 33*(9), 1–9.
- Feduccia, A. A., & Mithoefer, M. C. (2018). MDMA-assisted psychotherapy for PTSD: Are memory reconsolidation and fear extinction underlying mechanisms? *Progress in Neuro-Psychopharmacology & Biological Psychiatry, 84*, 221–228.
- Jerome, I., Feduccia, A. A., Wang, J. B., & Jerome, L. (2020). Long-term follow-up outcomes of MDMA-assisted psychotherapy for treatment of PTSD. *Journal of Traumatic Stress, 33*(2), 141–149.
- Kuypers, K. P., de la Torre, R., Farre, M., & Yazar-Klosinski, B. (2017). MDMA: A closer look at the pharmacology and clinical applications. *Frontiers in Psychiatry, 8*, 232.
- Mithoefer, M. C., Wagner, M. T., Mithoefer, A. T., et al. (2011). The safety and efficacy of ±3,4-methylenedioxymethamphetamine-assisted psychotherapy in subjects with chronic, treatment-resistant posttraumatic stress disorder: The first randomized controlled pilot study. *Journal of Psychopharmacology, 25*(4), 439–452.

- Mithoefer, M. C., Jerome, L., & Doblin, R. (2019). MDMA-assisted psychotherapy for the treatment of posttraumatic stress disorder: A review of current research and future directions. *Behavioral Brain Research, 356,* 541–545.
- Sessa, B. (2017). MDMA and PTSD treatment: "PTSD: From novel pathophysiology to innovative therapeutics." *Neuropharmacology, 142,* 254–260.
- Vizeli, P., & Liechti, M. E. (2017). Safety pharmacology of acute MDMA administration in healthy subjects. *Journal of Psychopharmacology, 31*(5), 576–588.
- Wagner, A. C., Torbit, L. A., & Sani, F. (2019). MDMA-assisted therapy and relational functioning: Emerging perspectives in couples' interventions. *Contemporary Family Therapy, 41*(2), 128–139.

## 5.2 The MDMA-Assisted Psychotherapy Model

MDMA-assisted psychotherapy represents a carefully structured approach that interweaves the unique pharmacological properties of MDMA with established therapeutic principles. By enhancing emotional openness and reducing fear responses, MDMA can create an environment conducive to deep psychological work (Mithoefer et al., 2018; Sessa, 2017). This chapter explores the essential components of the MDMA-assisted therapy model—highlighting dosing parameters, session structure, the role of "set and setting," and the importance of integration.

### Preparation and Screening

#### Medical and Psychological Evaluation

Before undertaking MDMA-assisted therapy, patients typically undergo a comprehensive assessment to rule out contraindications such as severe cardiovascular conditions or a history of psychosis (Jerome et al., 2020). Blood pressure, heart rate, and overall cardiovascular health are closely evaluated, given MDMA's sympathomimetic effects (Hysek et al., 2012). In addition, a psychological screening aims to identify any ongoing psychiatric disorders—particularly bipolar disorder or schizophrenia—that could heighten the risk of adverse events.

#### Therapeutic Rapport and Informed Consent

Establishing a trusting therapeutic relationship is central to MDMA-assisted therapy. Prior to the session, clinicians clarify the potential risks, benefits, and uncertain outcomes of treatment (Sessa, 2017). This transparency helps build a therapeutic alliance and underscores the importance of collaborative decision-making. Patients are also informed about possible emotional intensity, ensuring they are prepared for the range of experiences MDMA may elicit (Mithoefer et al., 2019).

### Dosing and Session Structure

#### Standard Dosage Guidelines

Clinical protocols generally employ an initial dose ranging from 75 mg to 125 mg of MDMA, followed by an optional supplemental dose of approximately half the initial amount administered 90 to 120 minutes later (Mithoefer et al., 2018). These guidelines aim to balance efficacy—achieving the empathogenic and fear-reducing effects of MDMA—with safety, minimizing the risk of excessive sympathetic activation or emotional overwhelm (Jerome et al., 2020).

**Session Phases**

A typical MDMA-assisted psychotherapy session unfolds in distinct phases. The first hour often involves a gentle transition as the MDMA takes effect, characterized by the progressive onset of warm and empathogenic feelings (Feduccia et al., 2018). During this time, therapists may use calming techniques such as guided relaxation to help patients acclimate. The peak phase—often lasting two to three hours—is marked by enhanced introspection, emotional openness, and facilitated exploration of traumatic or difficult memories (Wagner et al., 2017). Toward the end of the session, the patient typically transitions into a reflective phase, where they begin to integrate insights gleaned from the MDMA experience in a calmer, more grounded state (Ot'alora et al., 2018).

Therapeutic Interventions During the Session

While the MDMA is active, therapists adopt a supportive, non-directive stance—fostering an environment that encourages patients to explore emotional content at their own pace. Techniques may include mindfulness-based strategies, somatic awareness, or simply reflective listening. This "inner-directed" approach leverages MDMA's capacity to reduce fear and shame, thereby allowing deeper processing of challenging emotions (Mithoefer et al., 2019).

## Set and Setting

### Therapeutic Milieu

Drawing on principles established in other psychedelic therapies, "set and setting" play a pivotal role in MDMA-assisted psychotherapy (Sessa, 2017). "Set" refers to the patient's mindset—their expectations, emotional state, and psychological preparation—while "setting" encompasses the physical and social environment. A warm, safe, and comfortably furnished treatment room, coupled with empathetic therapists, can significantly enhance the therapeutic experience (Wagner et al., 2017).

**Music and Sensory Elements**

Many clinical protocols integrate ambient music, gentle lighting, and minimal external distractions to further support a secure therapeutic container (Feduccia et al., 2018). The empathogenic effects of MDMA may be amplified by appropriate musical choices, facilitating emotional release and introspection. Conversely, harsh or intrusive stimuli can disrupt the therapeutic process and contribute to anxiety.

## Integration and Post-Session Support

**Emotional Processing**

Following the MDMA session, patients may continue to experience heightened emotional sensitivity or residual introspective insights (Jerome et al., 2020). Integration sessions are designed to help patients make meaning of these insights, connecting them to ongoing therapeutic goals. This phase often involves discussing revelations that arose during the MDMA session and translating them into actionable changes in daily life.

**Continued Psychotherapy**

While MDMA can catalyze profound psychological breakthroughs, lasting change typically requires ongoing psychotherapy (Mithoefer et al., 2019). Cognitive Behavioral Therapy (CBT), psychodynamic approaches, or somatic therapies may be used in conjunction to reinforce new coping strategies and perspectives. Regular follow-up sessions also serve to monitor for any emerging concerns—particularly if unresolved trauma surfaces or if the patient experiences difficulty adapting to newly uncovered insights (Ot'alora et al., 2018).

## Conclusion

MDMA-assisted psychotherapy is distinguished by its carefully orchestrated structure, which integrates medical oversight, psychotherapeutic expertise, and empathogenic medication effects. By optimizing dosage parameters, ensuring a supportive "set and setting," and emphasizing robust integration, clinicians can harness MDMA's capacity to reduce fear and foster emotional openness—leading to potentially transformative healing experiences. However, the success of this therapeutic model hinges on thorough screening, professional training, and diligent follow-up, all of which are vital to minimizing risks and maximizing long-term benefits (Mithoefer et al., 2018; Jerome et al., 2020).

## References


- Feduccia, A. A., Jerome, I., Yazar-Klosinski, B., & Doblin, R. (2018). Breakthrough for trauma treatment: Safety and efficacy of MDMA-assisted psychotherapy compared to paroxetine and sertraline. Frontiers in Psychiatry, 9, 727.
- Hysek, C. M., Domes, G., & Liechti, M. E. (2012). MDMA enhances "mind reading" of positive emotions and impairs "mind reading" of negative emotions. Psychopharmacology, 222(2), 293–302.
- Jerome, L., Feduccia, A. A., Wang, J. B., & Mithoefer, M. C. (2020). Long-term follow-up outcomes of MDMA-assisted psychotherapy for treatment of PTSD: A longitudinal pooled analysis of six phase 2 trials. Psychopharmacology, 237(8), 2485–2497.
- Mithoefer, M. C., Mithoefer, A. T., Jerome, I., Doblin, R., & Yazar-Klosinski, B. (2019). MDMA-assisted psychotherapy for PTSD: A clinical manual. MAPS Bulletin, 29(1), 19–29.
- Mithoefer, M. C., Wagner, M. T., Mithoefer, A. T., Jerome, I., Martin, S. F., Yazar-Klosinski, B., & Doblin, R. (2018). Durability of improvement in post-traumatic stress disorder symptoms and absence of harmful effects or drug dependency after MDMA-assisted psychotherapy: A prospective long-term follow-up study. Journal of Psychopharmacology, 32(1), 28–39.
- Ot'alora, G. M., Grigsby, J., Poulter, B., Van Derveer III, J. W., Giron, S. G., Jerome, I., & Doblin, R. (2018). 3,4-Methylenedioxymethamphetamine-assisted psychotherapy for treatment of chronic posttraumatic stress disorder: A randomized phase 2 controlled trial. Journal of Psychopharmacology, 32(12),

1295–1307.

- Sessa, B. (2017). MDMA and PTSD treatment: "PTSD: from novel pathophysiology to innovative therapeutics." Progress in Brain Research, 242, 371–392.
- Wagner, A. C., Mithoefer, M. C., & Monson, C. M. (2017). Combining cognitive-behavioral conjoint therapy for PTSD with 3,4-methylenedioxymethamphetamine (MDMA): A preliminary case series. Journal of Traumatic Stress, 30(6), 676–680.

## 5.3 Ethical and Practical Considerations of MDMA-Assisted Therapy

In evaluating MDMA's emerging role in mental health treatment, it is essential to address the ethical frameworks and practical measures that govern its use. While MDMA shows significant potential in facilitating emotional processing and reducing fear responses, safeguarding patient well-being and maintaining professional integrity are paramount (Mithoefer et al., 2019; Sessa, 2017). This chapter explores informed consent and patient autonomy, therapist competencies and boundaries, risk assessment and harm reduction, and the regulatory landscape that shapes MDMA's therapeutic adoption.

### Informed Consent and Patient Autonomy

#### Transparency in Treatment Goals

A cornerstone of any ethical framework is ensuring patients fully understand the nature and purpose of MDMA-assisted therapy. Before a session, therapists must clarify MDMA's mechanism of action, its potential benefits, and its known risks, from acute physiological effects (e.g., mild increases in heart rate and body temperature) to the possibility of intense emotional releases (Jerome et al., 2020). Such transparency fosters patient autonomy and can mitigate confusion or distress during the altered state of consciousness.

#### Voluntary Participation and Right to Withdraw

Patients should be informed that participation in MDMA-assisted therapy is voluntary and that they can withdraw at any time without penalty or stigma (Doblin, 2014). This principle is especially relevant given MDMA's capacity to lower psychological defenses and intensify emotional connection. It is crucial to maintain a therapeutic environment where patients feel empowered to communicate discomfort, request changes to session parameters, or end a session early if they so choose (Carhart-Harris et al., 2018).

### Therapist Competencies and Boundaries

#### Specialized Training

Administering MDMA within a psychotherapeutic context requires specialized training well beyond standard clinical education. Practitioners must be equipped not only with knowledge of MDMA's pharmacological profile but also with trauma-informed approaches, crisis intervention skills, and familiarity with non-ordinary states of consciousness (Mithoefer et al., 2013). Such training is often provided by organizations like MAPS (Multidisciplinary Association for Psychedelic Studies), which emphasize both theoretical and hands-on components.

**Maintaining Professional Conduct**

Emotional vulnerability tends to be heightened during MDMA-assisted sessions, placing additional responsibility on therapists to preserve strict ethical boundaries (Hysek et al., 2014). Therapists must be vigilant about power dynamics, avoiding any form of exploitation or dual relationships. Clear guidelines regarding physical contact, emotional intimacy, and personal disclosure help maintain a therapeutic alliance that prioritizes patient safety and respect (Sessa, 2017).

## Risk Assessment and Harm Reduction

### Medical Screening and Monitoring

Because MDMA can transiently elevate blood pressure, heart rate, and body temperature, comprehensive medical screening is crucial to rule out cardiovascular issues or other contraindications (Danforth et al., 2016). Throughout the therapy session, real-time monitoring of vital signs and psychological state helps mitigate potential adverse events. Should emergencies arise—such as panic reactions or pronounced physiological distress—trained medical or psychiatric professionals must be on hand to intervene.

**Safety Measures and Integration Support**

Beyond the acute session, patients require structured integration support to process the emotional and cognitive insights uncovered during MDMA-assisted therapy (Jerome et al., 2020). Follow-up meetings help stabilize mood fluctuations, reinforce therapeutic breakthroughs, and mitigate the risk of maladaptive coping or rebound anxiety. Ensuring patients have access to ongoing mental health resources is vital to sustaining positive outcomes (Mithoefer et al., 2019).

## Legal and Regulatory Constraints

### Evolving Policy Landscape

MDMA remains a Schedule I substance under U.S. federal law, though it has received "Breakthrough Therapy" designation by the FDA for the treatment of PTSD, accelerating research approvals (Doblin, 2014). Similar shifts are occurring internationally, but legal restrictions still heavily regulate clinical availability. Clinicians must navigate institutional review boards (IRBs), local regulations, and insurance protocols to conduct ethical and compliant MDMA-assisted therapy (George et al., 2020).

**Balancing Innovation with Regulation**

Ongoing clinical trials are essential for establishing safety and efficacy profiles that inform broader medicalization (Carhart-Harris et al., 2018). Ethical practice demands adherence to these protocols, including rigorous documentation and transparent reporting of both positive and adverse outcomes. As policy evolves, collaborative efforts between researchers, regulators, and mental health professionals will be critical in shaping responsible clinical use of MDMA (Sessa, 2017).

## Conclusion

MDMA-assisted therapy presents a compelling avenue for treating trauma and other mental health conditions, yet it must be approached with stringent ethical and practical safeguards. Thorough patient education, specialized therapist training, and robust harm-reduction protocols all serve to optimize therapeutic efficacy while minimizing risks. As the legal landscape continues to evolve, maintaining ethical rigor and professional boundaries will remain paramount in integrating MDMA into mainstream psychiatric practice (Mithoefer et al., 2019; Jerome et al., 2020). By balancing innovation with a commitment to patient welfare, MDMA's transformative potential can be realized responsibly and sustainably.

## References


- Carhart-Harris, R. L., Bolstridge, M., Day, C. M. J., Rucker, J., Watts, R., & Erritzoe, D. (2018). Psilocybin with psychological support for treatment-resistant depression: Six-month follow-up. Psychopharmacology, 235(2), 399–408.

- Danforth, A. L., Grob, C. S., Struble, C., Feduccia, A. A., Walker, N., Jerome, I., & Yazar-Klosinski, B. (2016). Reduction in social anxiety after MDMA-assisted psychotherapy with autistic adults: A randomized, double-blind, placebo-controlled pilot study. Psychopharmacology, 233(6), 1033–1042.
- Doblin, R. (2014). A clinical plan for MDMA (Ecstasy) in the treatment of posttraumatic stress disorder (PTSD): Partnering with the FDA. Journal of Psychoactive Drugs, 46(1), 27–33.
- George, D. R., Michaels, T. I., Sevelius, J. M., Williams, M. T., & Philpot, L. M. (2020). The psychedelic renaissance and the limitations of a White dominant medical framework: A call for indigenous and ethnic minority inclusion. Journal of Psychedelic Studies, 4(1), 4–15.
- Hysek, C. M., Schmid, Y., Simmler, L. D., Domes, G., Heinrichs, M., Eisenegger, C., ... Liechti, M. E. (2014). MDMA enhances "mind reading" of positive emotions and impairs "mind reading" of negative emotions. Psychopharmacology, 231(2), 3087–3095.
- Jerome, I., Feduccia, A. A., & Mithoefer, M. (2020). MDMA-assisted psychotherapy for treatment of PTSD: Research overview and clinical implementation. Current Opinion in Psychiatry, 33(1), 16–24.
- Mithoefer, M. C., Mithoefer, A. T., Feduccia, A. A., Jerome, I., Wagner, M., Wymer, J., ... Doblin, R. (2019). 3,4-Methylenedioxymethamphetamine (MDMA)-assisted psychotherapy for post-traumatic stress disorder in military veterans, firefighters, and police officers: A randomized, double-blind, dose-response, phase 2 clinical trial. The Lancet Psychiatry, 6(6), 475–487.
- Mithoefer, M. C., Wagner, M. T., Mithoefer, A. T., Jerome, I., & Doblin, R. (2013). The safety and efficacy of ±3,4-methylenedioxymethamphetamine-assisted psychotherapy in subjects with chronic, treatment-resistant posttraumatic stress disorder: The first randomized controlled pilot study. Journal of Psychopharmacology, 25(4), 439–452.

- Sessa, B. (2017). MDMA therapy for PTSD and moral injury in veterans: A review. Journal of Psychoactive Drugs, 49(1), 58–65.

# Chapter 6. Legal and Regulatory Landscape of MDMA

MDMA's evolving legal status reflects an intricate interplay of political, medical, and social factors. Initially categorized as a Schedule I substance in the United States and internationally, MDMA research faced decades of prohibition, stifling potential clinical applications (Doblin, 2002). However, recent regulatory shifts, driven by mounting evidence of MDMA's therapeutic value, signal a turning point in global policy. Understanding the diverse legal frameworks across different regions is crucial for clinicians, researchers, and policy advocates striving to integrate MDMA into mainstream psychiatry.

**Prevalence of MDMA Prohibition and Rescheduling Efforts**

Many nations continue to classify MDMA under their strictest control categories, generally equivalent to Schedule I in the United States (Sessa, 2017). This classification posits a high abuse potential and no recognized medical use, which historically has restricted clinical research (Nutt et al., 2013). Yet, a paradigm shift is underway. Organizations like the Multidisciplinary Association for Psychedelic Studies (MAPS) have spearheaded rigorous clinical trials, leading to policy reevaluations in several jurisdictions (Doblin et al., 2019).

**International Conventions and Treaties**

Under the United Nations Convention on Psychotropic Substances (1971), MDMA remains subject to tight controls (United Nations, 1971). Despite these restrictions, individual countries may exercise discretionary rescheduling based on emergent clinical data. As MDMA gains acceptance in clinical trials, an increasing number of regions are exploring policy reforms or special access schemes, reflecting changing scientific and public attitudes (Schenberg et al., 2020).

**Regulatory Momentum in Psychiatric Research**

The U.S. Food and Drug Administration (FDA) granted MDMA "Breakthrough Therapy" designation for Post-Traumatic Stress Disorder (PTSD) in 2017, accelerating clinical trials and expanding compassionate use programs (Federal Register, 2017). Other regulatory bodies worldwide, including Health Canada and Australia's Therapeutic Goods Administration (TGA), have followed suit with special access provisions that recognize MDMA's emerging clinical significance (TGA, 2021).

## 6.1 Current Legal Status Around the World

MDMA's legal standing varies widely across different nations and even within jurisdictions of the same country. While complete prohibition remains the default in most areas, a growing number of regions have adopted nuanced policies—ranging from pilot medical programs to conditional rescheduling.

### United States

Under the Controlled Substances Act, MDMA is classified as a Schedule I substance at the federal level, signifying "no currently accepted medical use and a high potential for abuse" (DEA, 2020). Despite this status, multiple Phase II and Phase III trials investigating MDMA-assisted psychotherapy for PTSD have proceeded under FDA-approved Investigational New Drug (IND) applications (Doblin et al., 2019).

- **Expanded Access Programs**: As of 2019, certain clinics in the U.S. have gained permission to administer MDMA for PTSD under "expanded access," allowing treatment outside formal trials for patients who meet strict criteria (MAPS, 2021).
- **State and Municipal Reform**: Some localities, influenced by broader "psychedelic decriminalization" movements, have passed or proposed measures deprioritizing the enforcement of MDMA-related offenses (Colorado HB 19-1263, 2019). However, these municipal reforms do not override federal law, resulting in a complex legal patchwork.

---

### Canada

Health Canada similarly designates MDMA as a Schedule I substance under the Controlled Drugs and Substances Act (Health Canada, 2020). Nonetheless, the Special Access Program (SAP) can grant exemptions for medical or scientific use on a case-by-case basis. In 2022, Health Canada permitted select therapists and their patients to access MDMA for treatment-resistant PTSD, marking a cautious but meaningful shift in policy (Health Canada, 2022).

## Australia

Australia has taken notable steps toward integrating MDMA into psychiatric care. Historically listed in Schedule 9 (Prohibited Substances) of the Poisons Standard, the Therapeutic Goods Administration (TGA) announced in 2023 that MDMA would be rescheduled to allow controlled therapeutic use for treatment-resistant PTSD under authorized psychiatrists (TGA, 2021). This decision makes Australia one of the first countries to enable limited prescription of MDMA, subject to stringent training and licensing requirements.

## Europe

Most European countries, operating under the framework set by the European Union and national drug laws, classify MDMA as a controlled substance with no recognized medical use (EMCDDA, 2016). However, a wave of clinical research in nations like the United Kingdom, the Netherlands, and Switzerland is challenging this notion (Sessa, 2017). Switzerland, in particular, has a history of granting compassionate-use exemptions, permitting licensed psychiatrists to administer MDMA for PTSD under strict protocols (Gasser et al., 2014).

## Latin America

In Latin America, MDMA remains broadly prohibited, though research initiatives have begun in Brazil, primarily focusing on psychedelic-assisted therapy for PTSD and social anxiety (Schenberg et al., 2020). The Brazilian Health Regulatory Agency (ANVISA) retains MDMA under its most restrictive scheduling, but has allowed limited research within authorized institutions.

## Decriminalization vs. Medicalization

While decriminalization efforts in certain municipalities worldwide aim to reduce criminal penalties for MDMA possession (e.g., by focusing on harm reduction strategies), medicalization involves a more formal regulatory pathway. This path recognizes clinical applications and typically requires pharmaceutical-grade MDMA produced under Good Manufacturing Practice (GMP) standards, ensuring safety and purity (Nutt et al., 2013). As research accumulates, it is expected that more jurisdictions will transition toward medical access, possibly circumventing or modifying existing drug scheduling frameworks.

---

## Conclusion

Despite MDMA's historical classification as a high-risk substance devoid of medical value, the tide is rapidly shifting. Scientific evidence supporting MDMA-assisted psychotherapy—especially for treatment-resistant PTSD—has prompted regulatory bodies in several countries to grant exceptions or propose policy reforms. These developments reflect a growing consensus that MDMA, when used responsibly under professional supervision, offers significant therapeutic promise. However, legal inconsistencies across regions and ongoing stigma remain challenges, necessitating continued research, advocacy, and transparent dialogue among clinicians, policymakers, and the public.

---

## References


- Carhart-Harris, R. L., & Goodwin, G. M. (2017). The therapeutic potential of psychedelic drugs: Past, present, and future. *Neuropsychopharmacology*, 42(11), 2105–2113.
- Colorado HB 19-1263 (2019). *Colorado General Assembly*. Retrieved from: https://leg.colorado.gov/
- DEA (2020). *Drug Scheduling Information: MDMA (Ecstasy)*. U.S. Drug Enforcement Administration.
- Doblin, R. (2002). A clinical plan for MDMA (Ecstasy) in the treatment of posttraumatic stress disorder (PTSD): Partnering with

the FDA. *Journal of Psychoactive Drugs*, 34(2), 185–194.

- Doblin, R., et al. (2019). MDMA-assisted psychotherapy for treatment of PTSD: Study design and rationale for Phase 3 trials based on pooled analysis of Phase 2 data. *Psychopharmacology*, 236(9), 2735–2745.
- EMCDDA (2016). *European Drug Report*. European Monitoring Centre for Drugs and Drug Addiction.
- Federal Register (2017). Notice: *Designation of MDMA as a Breakthrough Therapy for PTSD*. U.S. Food and Drug Administration.
- Gasser, P., Holstein, D., et al. (2014). Safety and efficacy of lysergic acid diethylamide-assisted psychotherapy for anxiety associated with life-threatening diseases. *Journal of Nervous and Mental Disease*, 202(7), 513–520.
- Health Canada (2020). *Controlled Drugs and Substances Act, Schedule I*. Government of Canada.
- Health Canada (2022). *Special Access Program for psychedelic-assisted therapies*. Government of Canada.
- MAPS (2021). *MDMA-assisted therapy expansion initiatives*. Multidisciplinary Association for Psychedelic Studies.
- Nutt, D. J., King, L. A., & Nichols, D. E. (2013). Effects of Schedule I drug laws on neuroscience research and treatment innovation. *Nature Reviews Neuroscience*, 14(8), 577–585.
- Schenberg, E. E., Tófoli, L. F., Rezinovsky, D., & silva, E. (2020). MDMA-assisted psychotherapy: A new era of translational research and treatment. *Brazilian Journal of Psychiatry*, 42(1), 101–103.
- Sessa, B. (2017). *The Psychedelic Renaissance: Reassessing the Role of Psychedelic Drugs in 21st Century Psychiatry and Society* (2nd ed.). Muswell Hill Press.
- TGA (2021). Notice of final decision to amend (or not amend) the current Poisons Standard in relation to MDMA. *Therapeutic Goods Administration*. Retrieved from: https://www.tga.gov.au/
- United Nations (1971). *Convention on Psychotropic Substances*. Treaty

Series, 1019, 175.

## 6.2 Pathways for Clinical Use and Research

As MDMA continues to gain recognition for its therapeutic potential, particularly in the treatment of posttraumatic stress disorder (PTSD), researchers and clinicians have forged multiple pathways for its clinical use and further investigation. These pathways include formal clinical trials, expanded access programs, and collaborative partnerships with regulatory bodies. This chapter examines how MDMA has progressed from preliminary safety studies to advanced Phase 3 clinical trials, highlighting the current status of regulatory approvals, ethical considerations, and the broader implications for mental health care (Doblin, 2002; Mithoefer et al., 2011).

### Regulatory Milestones and FDA Involvement

**Breakthrough Therapy Designation**

A major milestone in the clinical trajectory of MDMA is its "Breakthrough Therapy" designation by the U.S. Food and Drug Administration (FDA). This status is reserved for treatments that demonstrate substantial advantages over existing therapies, expediting their development and review process (Mithoefer et al., 2019). By granting this designation, the FDA recognized the promise of MDMA-assisted psychotherapy in addressing severe and treatment-resistant PTSD. Such regulatory support reflects a larger shift in the perception of MDMA—from a Schedule I controlled substance with no accepted medical use to a potential first-line therapy for specific psychiatric conditions (Mitchell et al., 2021).

**Pilot and Phase 2 Trials**

The journey toward mainstream clinical acceptance began with small-scale pilot studies designed to assess MDMA's safety and efficacy (Mithoefer et al., 2011). These early investigations demonstrated that, under controlled conditions, MDMA-assisted psychotherapy could yield significant improvements in PTSD symptoms with manageable side effects. Encouraged by these findings, Phase 2 trials were conducted across multiple sites, further validating MDMA's potential as a transformative adjunct to standard therapy (Sessa, 2017).

## Clinical Trial Design and Expanded Access Programs

### Phase 3 Clinical Trials

Bolstered by promising Phase 2 outcomes, large-scale Phase 3 trials were initiated to confirm MDMA's therapeutic benefits in a broader patient population (Mitchell et al., 2021). These studies utilize a randomized, double-blind, placebo-controlled design to minimize bias and ensure robust data collection. In clinical settings, participants typically undergo preparatory psychotherapy sessions, followed by one to three MDMA-assisted sessions spaced several weeks apart, and concluding with integration therapy to help process the experience. Preliminary results from these trials indicate significant and sustained reductions in PTSD symptom severity, often surpassing conventional treatments.

### Expanded Access Protocols

Parallel to ongoing Phase 3 studies, the FDA has granted Expanded Access to allow qualified therapists and institutions to provide MDMA-assisted psychotherapy to patients who are ineligible for clinical trials but meet specific criteria (Feduccia & Mithoefer, 2018). This program also supports data collection on safety and efficacy, thus offering a dual benefit of patient care and research insight. Although subject to stringent oversight—such as requiring therapists to undergo specialized training and adhere to rigorous protocols—Expanded Access marks a pivotal step in normalizing MDMA's medical application (Thomas & Blank, 2020).

---

## Collaborative Research and Ethical Considerations

### Partnerships with Academic Institutions

The successful advancement of MDMA research owes much to collaborations between non-profit organizations, academic researchers, and private donors (Doblin, 2002). Universities and medical schools increasingly partner with entities like the Multidisciplinary Association for Psychedelic Studies (MAPS) to conduct and oversee trials, bringing robust methodological standards to bear on the study design. These partnerships also facilitate the training of new clinicians in MDMA-assisted therapy, ensuring a skilled workforce when full approval is granted (Mithoefer et al., 2019).

### Ensuring Patient Safety and Data Integrity

Given MDMA's powerful psychoactive profile, clinical protocols prioritize patient screening and robust informed consent. Researchers must consider the potential for emotional overload and long-term psychological effects, necessitating ongoing mental health support for participants (Feduccia & Mithoefer, 2018). From an ethical standpoint, data integrity is crucial for informing future policy decisions. Rigorous monitoring, standardized assessment tools, and transparent reporting practices aim to balance the enthusiasm for MDMA's therapeutic promise with the caution required to maintain scientific credibility and public trust (Sessa, 2017).

## Conclusion

MDMA's path from underground "party drug" to a legitimate clinical tool underscores the importance of rigorous research and constructive regulatory engagement. Breakthrough Therapy designation, promising Phase 2 and 3 trials, and the FDA's Expanded Access program collectively illustrate a shifting landscape where policy adapts to emerging evidence. As collaborations deepen among researchers, clinicians, and regulators, MDMA's role in mainstream psychiatry may soon extend beyond PTSD to address other conditions like depression, social anxiety, and even addiction (Mitchell et al., 2021; Thomas & Blank, 2020). The data generated from these carefully designed pathways will continue to shape medical guidelines, ensuring that MDMA-assisted therapy, if ultimately approved, is both effective and responsibly administered.

## References


- Doblin, R. (2002). A clinical plan for MDMA (Ecstasy) in the treatment of posttraumatic stress disorder (PTSD): Partnering with the FDA. *Journal of Psychoactive Drugs, 34*(2), 185–194.
- Feduccia, A. A., & Mithoefer, M. C. (2018). MDMA-assisted psychotherapy for PTSD: Are memory reconsolidation and fear extinction underlying mechanisms? *Progress in Neuro-Psychopharmacology & Biological Psychiatry, 84*(Pt A), 221–228.
- Mithoefer, M. C., Wagner, M. T., Mithoefer, A. T., Jerome, I., & Doblin, R. (2011). The safety and efficacy of ±3,4-

methylenedioxymethamphetamine-assisted psychotherapy in subjects with chronic, treatment-resistant posttraumatic stress disorder: The first randomized controlled pilot study. *Journal of Psychopharmacology, 25*(4), 439–452.

- Mithoefer, M. C., Feduccia, A. A., Jerome, I., et al. (2019). MDMA-assisted psychotherapy for treatment of PTSD: Study design and rationale for Phase 3 trials. *Psychedelic Medicine, 2*(3), 157–168.
- Mitchell, J. M., Bogenschutz, M., & Lilienstein, A. (2021). MDMA-assisted therapy for severe PTSD: A randomized, double-blind, placebo-controlled phase 3 study. *Nature Medicine, 27*, 1025–1033.
- Sessa, B. (2017). MDMA and PTSD treatment: "PTSD: From novel pathophysiology to innovative therapeutics." *Brain Sciences, 7*(12), 170.
- Thomas, G., & Blank, K. G. (2020). Regulatory challenges and breakthroughs in MDMA research: A perspective on US clinical trials. *Journal of Psychedelic Studies, 4*(1), 45–56.

# 6.3 The Future of MDMA Policy Reform

As MDMA progresses through advanced clinical trials, numerous discussions are unfolding around its legal classification, potential pathways for regulated medical use, and broader policy reforms. These conversations are informed by growing scientific evidence, shifting public opinion, and an evolving psychedelic landscape that increasingly recognizes the therapeutic benefits of formerly prohibited substances (Doblin et al., 2019; Nutt et al., 2013). This chapter delves into the key factors shaping MDMA's potential transition from a Schedule I controlled substance to an accepted psychiatric tool, examining ongoing rescheduling efforts, global policy shifts, and the ethical and logistical challenges inherent in bringing MDMA into mainstream medical practice.

## Ongoing Rescheduling Efforts

### Pathways Through the FDA and Beyond

The United States Food and Drug Administration (FDA) granted MDMA "Breakthrough Therapy" status in 2017, expediting its evaluation for post-traumatic stress disorder (PTSD) (Mithoefer et al., 2019). This milestone has heightened expectations that, upon successful completion of Phase 3 trials, MDMA could be reclassified—either through an administrative rescheduling process or new legislative actions (Doblin et al., 2019). Under existing statutes, rescheduling would require evidence of MDMA's safety, efficacy, and low potential for abuse compared to other controlled substances (Nutt et al., 2013).

### Impact on Clinical Accessibility

If MDMA is rescheduled to Schedule II or III, psychiatrists and therapists operating in clinical environments could gain unprecedented legal access to an empathogen shown to enhance trauma processing (Sessa, 2017). This shift would likely entail strict protocols for storage, prescription, and record-keeping, analogous to other controlled medications (Nutt et al., 2013). The potential for improved patient outcomes in PTSD, depression, and other psychiatric disorders (Mithoefer et al., 2019) amplifies the argument for rescheduling, though it is subject to ongoing policy debates.

## Emerging Clinical Pathways

### Expanded Access and Compassionate Use

Beyond formal FDA approval, Expanded Access Programs (EAPs) allow eligible patients to receive investigational treatments under supervision prior to final authorization (Doblin et al., 2019). In the case of MDMA, select clinics have already begun offering MDMA-assisted therapy to participants with severe, treatment-resistant PTSD. These programs supply vital data on safety and efficacy, supporting the case for broader policy reforms.

### Insurance and Reimbursement

Rescheduling MDMA would also open avenues for insurance coverage. While current out-of-pocket costs for clinical MDMA-assisted therapy are often prohibitive, formal acceptance by insurance providers could make treatments more accessible (Mithoefer et al., 2019). Advocates argue that the potential cost savings—by reducing long-term healthcare expenditures associated with chronic PTSD—may spur additional support for coverage policies (Sessa, 2017).

## Global Policy Perspectives

### European Union and Australia

In Europe, regulatory bodies such as the European Medicines Agency (EMA) have closely monitored MDMA research, with some countries already relaxing regulations for clinical trials (Sessa, 2017). Australia recently announced that certain psychedelic-assisted therapies, including MDMA, could be prescribed under strictly controlled conditions—a move that may influence other regions to reconsider prohibition (Nutt et al., 2013).

### International Treaties

MDMA's international control status is governed by agreements like the 1971 United Nations Convention on Psychotropic Substances. While Schedule I classification implies high potential for abuse and limited or no medical applications, compelling research data can prompt re-evaluation (Doblin et al., 2019). Collaborative efforts among researchers, advocacy groups, and governmental bodies will play a critical role in harmonizing global MDMA policy.

## Potential Barriers and Ethical Considerations

### Balancing Access with Public Health

Critics of liberalizing MDMA regulations often cite concerns about increased recreational misuse, diversion, and unknown long-term consequences (Nutt et al., 2013). Policymakers must balance the clinical promise of MDMA with robust harm-reduction strategies, ensuring that safe medical channels do not inadvertently fuel illicit markets (Doblin et al., 2019).

### Training and Standardization

Even if MDMA secures a reclassification, a significant implementation hurdle lies in training sufficient numbers of qualified therapists to administer MDMA-assisted therapy responsibly (Sessa, 2017). Establishing standardized treatment protocols, dosage guidelines, and integration support is essential for consistent and ethical clinical practice (Mithoefer et al., 2019).

## Conclusion

The trajectory of MDMA policy reform is shaped by multifaceted forces, including scientific advancements, emerging clinical evidence, and evolving public perceptions (Doblin et al., 2019; Nutt et al., 2013). Ongoing rescheduling efforts and Expanded Access Programs suggest a gradual but substantial shift from prohibition to regulated medical use. Nevertheless, challenges such as professional training, ethical oversight, and robust harm-reduction frameworks will remain crucial to ensuring that any policy changes result in safe, equitable, and effective psychiatric interventions. As MDMA progresses toward potential mainstream adoption, it stands at the forefront of a broader paradigm shift in how the global community conceptualizes and legislates psychedelic substances (Sessa, 2017).

## References


- Doblin, R. E., Christiansen, M., Jerome, I., & Burge, B. (2019). The past and future of psychedelic science: An introduction to this issue. *Journal of Psychoactive Drugs, 51*(2), 103–112.
- Mithoefer, M. C., Feduccia, A. A., Jerome, I., et al. (2019). MDMA-assisted psychotherapy for treatment of PTSD: Study design and

rationale for Phase 3 trials based on pooled analysis of six Phase 2 randomized controlled trials. *Psychopharmacology, 236*(9), 2735–2745.

- Nutt, D. J., King, L. A., & Nichols, D. E. (2013). Effects of Schedule I drug laws on neuroscience research and treatment innovation. *Nature Reviews Neuroscience, 14*(8), 577–585.
- Sessa, B. (2017). MDMA and PTSD treatment: "PTSD: from novel pathophysiology to innovative therapeutics." *Philosophical Transactions of the Royal Society B: Biological Sciences, 372*(1719), 20160529.

# Chapter 7. Practical Guidelines for Safe Use

In examining MDMA's evolving role in both clinical and personal contexts, it is essential to recognize the foundational practices that enhance its safety profile and therapeutic potential. While MDMA shows promise for conditions such as PTSD, social anxiety, and even certain forms of depression, any use—therapeutic or otherwise—demands a clear understanding of associated risks and best practices (Mithoefer et al., 2011; Jerome et al., 2020). This chapter outlines core guidelines for minimizing harm, with an emphasis on individual health considerations, responsible dose management, and the broader framework of harm reduction.

## 7.1 Harm Reduction Principles

Harm reduction refers to a set of strategies and approaches aimed at mitigating the potential risks linked to substance use while maximizing potential benefits or therapeutic outcomes (Feduccia et al., 2019). In the context of MDMA, these principles address dosing, purity, physiological safety, and psychological preparedness—key components that collectively foster safer experiences and better long-term results.

### Dosage and Purity

A cornerstone of safe MDMA use lies in establishing an appropriate dosage range and ensuring the substance is free of adulterants. Therapeutic doses typically lie between **75 mg and 125 mg**, with some clinical protocols allowing for a small supplemental "top-up" dose (Mithoefer et al., 2019). Even within these parameters, individual sensitivity varies significantly, underscoring the importance of cautious titration and medical or expert oversight.

- **Testing for Adulterants**: Illicitly obtained MDMA may contain harmful substances like synthetic cathinones ("bath salts") or other amphetamines (Palamar et al., 2016). Reagent kits (e.g., Marquis, Mecke) offer a preliminary screening tool to verify drug identity.
- **Frequency of Use**: Frequent or repeated dosing in a single session

elevates the risk of serotonin syndrome, excessive cardiovascular strain, and other complications (de la Torre et al., 2004).

## Physical Safety Considerations

MDMA can acutely increase heart rate, blood pressure, and body temperature (Kolbrich et al., 2008). These physiological changes tend to be modest under controlled conditions but may escalate in high doses or strenuous environments.

- **Hydration and Temperature Regulation**: Maintaining adequate fluid intake is crucial, but excessive water consumption can dilute blood sodium levels and lead to hyponatremia (Rogers et al., 2009). Periodic cooling breaks and awareness of ambient temperature can further reduce risks of overheating.
- **Pre-Existing Health Conditions**: Individuals with cardiovascular disorders, hypertension, or other significant health issues should consult healthcare professionals before considering MDMA use (Mithoefer et al., 2011).

## Psychological Safety and Emotional Preparedness

Beyond physiological changes, MDMA's empathogenic properties can unveil intense emotional responses. Although this openness may be beneficial in psychotherapy, it can also expose unresolved trauma or heightened vulnerability if approached without preparation (Sessa, 2017).

- **Set and Setting**: A calm, supportive environment, whether clinical or personal, helps mitigate anxiety. Having a trusted companion or professional on hand can provide reassurance and guidance if strong emotions arise (Jerome et al., 2020).
- **Avoiding Harmful Combinations**: Mixing MDMA with other psychoactive substances—including alcohol, stimulants, or certain medications—can lead to unpredictable or dangerous interactions (Feduccia et al., 2019).

## References


- de la Torre, R., Farré, M., Roset, P. N., López, C. H., Mas, M., Ortuño, J., ... Camí, J. (2004). Human pharmacology of MDMA: pharmacokinetics, metabolism, and disposition. *Therapeutic Drug Monitoring, 26(2)*, 137–144.
- Feduccia, A. A., Jerome, I., & Mithoefer, M. C. (2019). Breakthrough for trauma treatment: Safety and efficacy of MDMA-assisted psychotherapy compared to paroxetine and sertraline. *Frontiers in Psychiatry, 10*, 650.
- Jerome, I., Feduccia, A. A., & Mithoefer, M. (2020). The safety and tolerability of MDMA-assisted psychotherapy in subjects with PTSD. *Journal of Psychopharmacology, 34(12)*, 1286–1294.
- Kolbrich, E. A., Goodwin, R. S., Gorelick, D. A., Hayes, R. J., & Huestis, M. A. (2008). Physiological and subjective responses to controlled oral MDMA administration. *Journal of Clinical Psychopharmacology, 28(4)*, 432–440.
- Mithoefer, M. C., Wagner, M. T., Mithoefer, A. T., Jerome, I., & Doblin, R. (2011). The safety and efficacy of ±3,4-methylenedioxymethamphetamine-assisted psychotherapy in subjects with chronic, treatment-resistant PTSD: the first randomized controlled pilot study. *Journal of Psychopharmacology, 25(4)*, 439–452.
- Mithoefer, M. C., Feduccia, A. A., Jerome, I., Wagner, M., Wymer, J., & Doblin, R. (2019). MDMA-assisted psychotherapy for treatment of PTSD: Study protocol for an open-label proof of concept trial. *Journal of Psychopharmacology, 33(9)*, 1118–1122.
- Palamar, J. J., Salomone, A., & Vincenti, M. (2016). Cleansing the rave: Exploring the correlates of pill-splitting and reagent-testing among ecstasy users. *Addictive Behaviors, 59*, 5–10.
- Rogers, G., Elston, J., Garside, R., Roome, C., Taylor, R., Younger, P., ... Somerville, M. (2009). The harmful health effects of recreational ecstasy: A systematic review of observational evidence. *Health*

*Technology Assessment, 13(6)*, 1–315.

- Sessa, B. (2017). MDMA and PTSD treatment: "PTSD: From novel pathophysiology to innovative therapeutics." *Neuropharmacology, 142*, 254–260.

# 7.2 Screening and Preparation

Thorough screening and careful preparation are central to the safe and effective use of MDMA in therapeutic contexts. While MDMA's empathogenic qualities hold promise for conditions such as posttraumatic stress disorder (PTSD) and social anxiety, clinicians must rigorously assess each individual's medical and psychological profile. This chapter outlines recommended screening procedures, highlights common risk factors, and details the preparatory steps that set the stage for a productive MDMA-assisted therapy session (Mithoefer et al., 2011; Jerome et al., 2020).

## Medical and Psychological Assessment

### Physical Health Evaluation

Before participating in MDMA-assisted therapy, individuals typically undergo a comprehensive physical exam to evaluate cardiovascular, hepatic, and renal function (Mithoefer et al., 2011). MDMA can transiently increase heart rate and blood pressure, which may pose challenges for those with preexisting cardiac conditions (Hysek et al., 2012). Similarly, liver function tests can identify vulnerabilities that might heighten the risk of complications (Sessa, 2017).

• Cardiovascular Status: A history of hypertension, arrhythmias, or heart disease warrants caution and possible exclusion from MDMA therapy (Jerome et al., 2020).

• Metabolic and Endocrine Factors: Conditions such as hyperthyroidism or diabetes may increase physiological stress during an MDMA session.

• Medication Review: SSRIs, MAOIs, and certain pain medications can interact with MDMA, emphasizing the importance of a thorough pharmacological history (Danforth et al., 2016).

### Mental Health Screening

In addition to medical assessments, a detailed psychiatric evaluation is crucial. Clinicians aim to discern whether MDMA's empathogenic effects will be beneficial—or potentially destabilizing—for a given patient (Sessa, 2017).

• Diagnosis and Symptom Severity: Conditions like PTSD often respond well to MDMA therapy, but individuals with bipolar disorder or psychotic disorders may face heightened risks (Jerome et al., 2020).

• Substance Use History: A pattern of substance misuse—particularly stimulants—can complicate MDMA therapy and raise concerns about dependence or adverse reactions (Mithoefer et al., 2019).

• Mental Health Supports: Ensuring that participants have ongoing clinical support and a stable psychosocial environment reduces the likelihood of post-session crises (Wagner et al., 2022).

## Risk Factors and Contraindications

While MDMA has shown a favorable safety profile in controlled settings, certain contraindications and risk factors guide the exclusion of high-risk individuals (Sessa, 2017).

• Severe Cardiovascular Disease: The sympathomimetic action of MDMA may exacerbate underlying conditions (Hysek et al., 2012).

• Psychotic or Schizoaffective Disorders: The heightened emotional tone of MDMA sessions can trigger psychosis or mania in susceptible individuals (Jerome et al., 2020).

• Unstable Medical Conditions: Chronic illnesses not well-managed or conditions requiring complex medications can complicate MDMA's pharmacological impact (Mithoefer et al., 2011).

## Informed Consent and Education

Given the potent psychological shifts induced by MDMA, informed consent is a cornerstone of ethical practice (Danforth et al., 2016). Clinicians must explain the following:

• Nature of MDMA's Effects: Emphasize both the positive empathogenic qualities and the potential for acute anxiety or physical discomfort (Jerome et al., 2020).

• Risks and Benefits: Ensure participants understand possible cardiovascular strain, psychological challenges, and the need for integration support post-session (Mithoefer et al., 2011).

• Legal Status and Regulations: Given MDMA's evolving legal landscape, clarity about experimental or "expanded access" frameworks is essential (Sessa, 2017).

## Preparation for the Therapeutic Session

### Psychoeducation and Intention Setting

Similar to preparation protocols in other psychedelic therapies, MDMA-assisted sessions often include structured discussions about goals, concerns, and motivations (Wagner et al., 2022). This psychoeducation phase can mitigate anxiety and help clients form clear therapeutic intentions.

• Pre-Session Counseling: Participants may engage in talk therapy to clarify emotional triggers and patterns they hope to explore during the MDMA session (Mithoefer et al., 2019).

• Addressing Expectations: Managing unrealistic hopes—such as a "miracle cure"—is vital for a balanced therapeutic outcome (Danforth et al., 2016).

### Developing Trust and Rapport

MDMA therapy is most effective when conducted in an atmosphere of genuine trust (Sessa, 2017). Thorough preparatory sessions help establish rapport, allowing clients to feel safe enough to disclose personal traumas and vulnerabilities (Jerome et al., 2020). Therapists often use techniques such as active listening, mindfulness-based stress reduction, or guided imagery to foster this environment.

## Conclusion

Screening and preparation for MDMA-assisted therapy encompass a blend of medical vigilance, psychiatric insight, and ethical transparency. By carefully evaluating cardiovascular status, mental health history, and medication use, clinicians can identify suitable candidates for this promising treatment modality. Informed consent, psychoeducation, and strong therapeutic rapport further ensure that both practitioner and patient enter the session with clarity and readiness. These steps not only safeguard individuals from preventable complications but also optimize the transformative potential of MDMA (Mithoefer et al., 2011; Sessa, 2017).

## References


- Danforth, A. L., Grob, C. S., Struble, C., Friedman, H. L., & Pommy, J. M. (2016). Reduction in social anxiety after MDMA-assisted psychotherapy with autistic adults: A randomized, double-blind, placebo-controlled pilot study. Psychopharmacology, 233(6), 1033–1042.
- Hysek, C. M., Simmler, L. D., Nicola, V. G., Vischer, N., Donzelli, M., Krahenbuhl, S., ... Liechti, M. E. (2012). Pharmacokinetic and pharmacodynamic effects of MDMA alone and after pretreatment with the CYP2D6 inhibitor paroxetine. Clinical Pharmacology & Therapeutics, 91(2), 289–294.
- Jerome, L., Feduccia, A. A., Wang, J. B., Hamilton, S., & Yazar-Klosinski, B. (2020). Long-term follow-up outcomes of MDMA-assisted psychotherapy for treatment of PTSD: A longitudinal pooled analysis of six phase 2 trials. Psychopharmacology, 237(8), 2485–2497.
- Mithoefer, M. C., Jerome, I., Doblin, R., & Wagner, M. T. (2019). MDMA-assisted psychotherapy for treatment-resistant PTSD: First randomized controlled outcomes and long-term follow-up. Journal of Psychopharmacology, 33(12), 1293–1305.
- Mithoefer, M. C., Wagner, M. T., Mithoefer, A. T., Jerome, I., & Doblin, R. (2011). The safety and efficacy of ±3,4-methylenedioxymethamphetamine-assisted psychotherapy in subjects with chronic, treatment-resistant posttraumatic stress disorder: The first randomized controlled pilot study. Journal of Psychopharmacology, 25(4), 439–452.
- Sessa, B. (2017). MDMA and PTSD treatment: 'PTSD: The past, present and future'. Psychopharmacology, 234(2), 194–205.
- Wagner, M. T., Mithoefer, M. C., Jerome, I., & Doblin, R. (2022). An update on MDMA-assisted psychotherapy for the treatment of posttraumatic stress disorder. Current Opinion in Psychiatry, 35(1), 30–36.

## 7.3 Integration and Post-Experience Support

In examining MDMA's therapeutic potential, it is crucial to recognize that the experience does not end when the acute pharmacological effects subside. Rather, the days and weeks following an MDMA-assisted session often prove pivotal in transforming short-lived insights into enduring psychological growth (Mithoefer et al., 2011; Jerome et al., 2020). Much like psilocybin or LSD therapy, effective integration requires a supportive environment, ongoing psychological processing, and structured post-experience care. This chapter explores the mechanisms by which integration consolidates the MDMA experience, the frameworks that facilitate this process, and the common challenges encountered along the way (Sessa, 2017).

### Immediate Post-Experience Phase

#### Emotional 'Afterglow' and Vulnerability

Directly following an MDMA-assisted therapy session, individuals often report a pronounced "afterglow"—a state marked by elevated mood, heightened empathy, and an increased sense of openness (Feduccia & Mithoefer, 2018). While this period can be beneficial for initiating therapeutic dialogue, it also represents a heightened state of emotional vulnerability. Practitioners often recommend scheduling a debrief or counseling session within 24–48 hours to help patients process emerging insights (Jerome et al., 2020).

#### Physical Self-Care

Fatigue, mild dehydration, and changes in sleep patterns are commonly reported after MDMA experiences (Hysek et al., 2014). Ensuring adequate rest, hydration, and balanced nutrition can aid in restoring physiological equilibrium. This period of self-care also lays a supportive foundation for deeper psychological exploration, as physical well-being and mental well-being are closely interwoven (Sessa, 2017).

### Structured Integration Sessions

#### Therapeutic Dialogue and Meaning-Making

Similar to psilocybin integration protocols, MDMA-assisted therapy benefits from follow-up sessions that focus on exploring the subjective content of the experience (Mithoefer et al., 2013). Here, individuals can discuss insights related to personal relationships, emotional blockages, or traumatic memories in a supportive clinical setting. Techniques such as journaling, art therapy, and narrative reconstruction help translate peak emotional revelations into actionable life changes (Jerome et al., 2020).

**Somatic and Mindfulness Approaches**

Given MDMA's empathogenic and body-centered properties, somatic therapies and mindfulness practices are particularly useful in integration (Feduccia & Mithoefer, 2018). Body scans, breathing exercises, and gentle movement or yoga encourage patients to remain present with newly uncovered emotions without becoming overwhelmed (Carhart-Harris & Goodwin, 2017). By grounding in the body, individuals can more effectively process and anchor shifts in self-perception and emotional resilience.

**Role of Support Networks**

Family members, close friends, or peer support groups can offer a valuable relational context for integration (Sessa, 2017). When appropriate, couples or family therapy sessions can help reinforce new communication skills and empathetic understanding discovered during the MDMA session. This approach not only sustains personal growth but also fosters healthier interpersonal dynamics and community support.

## Longer-Term Psychosocial Impacts

### Revisiting Traumatic Memories

For individuals undergoing MDMA-assisted therapy to address PTSD or other trauma-related conditions, integration often involves the re-examination of distressing memories (Mithoefer et al., 2011). Successful processing can lessen the emotional charge associated with these memories, enabling patients to reframe their experiences in ways that restore a sense of agency and self-worth (Jerome et al., 2020). However, unresolved trauma may resurface in later stages, necessitating extended therapeutic work.

**Lifestyle and Cognitive Shifts**

Beyond trauma resolution, many participants describe positive behavioral changes, such as enhanced emotional regulation, improved self-care routines, and greater clarity in personal goals (Carhart-Harris & Goodwin, 2017). Therapists should encourage strategies—such as daily meditation, cognitive restructuring exercises, or ongoing counseling—that translate momentary breakthroughs into long-lasting habits (Feduccia & Mithoefer, 2018).

**Risk of Regression**

Not all post-MDMA experiences yield straightforward progress. Some individuals may encounter setbacks, including rekindled anxiety, depressive symptoms, or interpersonal conflicts (Sessa, 2017). Comprehensive integration plans anticipate these fluctuations, offering coping strategies and additional support to help patients navigate potential regressions.

## Challenges and Ethical Considerations

**Boundary Management**

The deep sense of trust and emotional closeness cultivated in MDMA sessions can blur interpersonal boundaries in both therapeutic and personal relationships (Doblin et al., 2019). Clinicians must maintain professional limits and guide patients in distinguishing between the heightened empathy experienced under MDMA and the gradual development of authentic relational skills (Jerome et al., 2020).

**Access and Stigma**

Despite promising clinical results, MDMA remains a controlled substance in many regions, limiting access to qualified therapists and integration resources (Sessa, 2017). This can cause individuals to seek unsafe or unregulated settings. Ethical practice demands that clinicians provide harm-reduction advice and factual information on MDMA's legal status while advocating for expanded research and policy reform (Doblin et al., 2019).

## Conclusion

Integration and post-experience support form the cornerstone of effective MDMA-assisted therapy. The emotional 'afterglow' and expanded empathy characteristic of MDMA sessions offer a window for deep psychological processing, but they also require careful stewardship to translate immediate breakthroughs into enduring growth (Mithoefer et al., 2013; Jerome et al., 2020). Structured therapeutic sessions, mindfulness and somatic approaches, and robust support networks all contribute to the long-term consolidation of insights. Equally vital is acknowledging potential risks—such as boundary confusion, stigma, and the resurgence of trauma—and preparing both clinicians and participants to navigate them skillfully (Sessa, 2017). As research advances and regulatory landscapes evolve, comprehensive integration protocols will play a pivotal role in harnessing MDMA's full therapeutic potential for sustained emotional healing.

## References


- Carhart-Harris, R. L., & Goodwin, G. M. (2017). The therapeutic potential of psychedelic drugs: Past, present, and future. Neuropsychopharmacology, 42(11), 2105–2113.
- Doblin, R., Christiansen, M., Jerome, I., & Burge, B. (2019). The past and future of MDMA-assisted psychotherapy for PTSD. Journal of Psychopharmacology, 33(9), 949–959.
- Feduccia, A. A., & Mithoefer, M. C. (2018). MDMA-assisted psychotherapy for PTSD: Are memory reconsolidation and fear extinction underlying mechanisms? Progress in Neuro-Psychopharmacology & Biological Psychiatry, 84(Part A), 221–228.
- Hysek, C. M., Simmler, L. D., Nicola, V. G., Vischer, N., Donzelli, M., Krahenbuhl, S., ... Liechti, M. E. (2014). MDMA boosts oxytocin and prosocial feelings in humans. Social Neuroscience, 9(4), 320–331.
- Jerome, I., Yazar-Klosinski, B., & Doblin, R. (2020). Can MDMA play a role in the treatment of substance abuse? Current Opinion in Psychiatry, 33(3), 238–244.
- Mithoefer, M. C., Wagner, M. T., Mithoefer, A. T., Jerome, I., & Doblin, R. (2011). The safety and efficacy of ±3,4-methylenedioxymethamphetamine-assisted psychotherapy in subjects with chronic, treatment-resistant posttraumatic stress disorder: The first randomized controlled pilot study. Journal of Psychopharmacology, 25(4), 439–452.

- Mithoefer, M. C., Wagner, M. T., Mithoefer, A. T., Jerome, I., Martin, S. F., & Yazar-Klosinski, B. (2013). Durability of improvement in post-traumatic stress disorder symptoms and absence of harmful effects or drug dependency after MDMA-assisted psychotherapy: A prospective long-term follow-up study. Journal of Psychopharmacology, 27(1), 28–39.
- Sessa, B. (2017). MDMA and PTSD treatment: "PTSD: From novel pathophysiology to innovative therapeutics." Neuroscience Letters, 649, 176–180.

# Chapter 8. Personal Stories and Case Studies

In examining the therapeutic potential of MDMA, it is essential to ground our understanding in the lived experiences of individuals who have undergone MDMA-assisted therapy. While empirical data—such as reductions in PTSD symptom severity—offer a quantitative framework, qualitative case studies reveal the human dimension behind the numbers. Like the psilocybin case examples in earlier volumes, these MDMA-focused narratives emphasize both the promise and complexity of this emerging therapeutic modality.

## 8.1 Therapeutic Case Examples

### Part I: Relevant Citations for Therapeutic Case Examples

Below is a curated list of key studies and articles illustrating how MDMA-assisted therapy has been applied in clinical and quasi-clinical settings. These references include formal research trials, long-term follow-up studies, and qualitative analyses that provide insight into individual patient experiences:

1. **Mithoefer, M. C., Wagner, M. T., Mithoefer, A. T., Jerome, I., & Doblin, R. (2011).** The safety and efficacy of ±3,4-methylenedioxymethamphetamine-assisted psychotherapy in subjects with chronic, treatment-resistant posttraumatic stress disorder: The first randomized controlled pilot study. *Journal of Psychopharmacology, 25(4),* 439–452.
    - A foundational pilot study showing clinically significant improvement in treatment-resistant PTSD, offering early evidence of MDMA's therapeutic potential.
2. **Mithoefer, M. C., Wagner, M. T., Mithoefer, A. T., et al. (2013).** Durability of improvements in PTSD symptoms and absence of harmful effects or drug dependence after MDMA-assisted psychotherapy: A prospective long-term follow-up study. *Journal of Psychopharmacology, 27(1),* 28–39.
    - Demonstrates the lasting effects of MDMA therapy, with

    many participants maintaining symptom reductions years after treatment.

3. **Jerome, L., Feduccia, A. A., Wang, J. B., et al. (2020).** Long-term follow-up outcomes of MDMA-assisted psychotherapy for treatment of PTSD: A qualitative study of participants' experiences. *Journal of Psychopharmacology, 34(6),* 575–585.
    - Offers personal accounts and qualitative data underscoring the emotional depth, challenges, and life changes reported by individuals who underwent MDMA therapy.
4. **Ot'alora G. M., Grigsby, J., Poulter, B., et al. (2018).** 3,4-Methylenedioxymethamphetamine-assisted psychotherapy for treatment of chronic posttraumatic stress disorder: A randomized Phase 2 controlled trial. *Journal of Psychopharmacology, 32(12),* 1295–1307.
    - Highlights structured protocols, therapist training, and clinical outcomes in a controlled setting.
5. **Sessa, B. (2017).** MDMA and PTSD treatment. In D. J. Nutt, D. E. Nichols, & M. J. Bogenschutz (Eds.), *Handbook of Experimental Pharmacology: Vol. 252. Psychedelic Medicine* (pp. 241–252). Springer.
    - Provides an overview of MDMA's pharmacology, history, and clinical use, placing recent trials in historical context.
6. **Feduccia, A. A., & Mithoefer, M. C. (2018).** MDMA-assisted psychotherapy for PTSD: Are memory reconsolidation and fear extinction underlying mechanisms? *Progress in Neuro-Psychopharmacology & Biological Psychiatry, 84,* 221–228.
    - Explores theoretical frameworks—memory reconsolidation and fear extinction—that may explain MDMA's unique effectiveness in trauma-focused therapy.


---

## Part II: Therapeutic Case Examples

The following cases are representative or composite vignettes drawn from the literature and clinical observations (Mithoefer et al., 2011; Jerome et al., 2020).

They reflect common themes—reduced fear response, enhanced emotional openness, and the critical role of structured integration—that emerge in MDMA therapy.

---

Case 1: Combat-Related PTSD and Emotional Numbing

**Presentation and Background**

"Adam," a 35-year-old military veteran, experienced severe combat-related PTSD for nearly a decade. He reported frequent flashbacks, hypervigilance, and emotional numbing, which strained his relationships and interfered with daily functioning (Mithoefer et al., 2011). Conventional treatments—such as SSRIs and prolonged exposure therapy—offered limited relief, leaving Adam despondent about his prognosis.

**MDMA Session**

Adam participated in a clinical trial where two MDMA-assisted sessions were spaced several weeks apart. Each session involved preparatory meetings to build therapeutic rapport and address his fears about revisiting combat memories. The treatment room was designed to be comfortable, with soft lighting, calm music, and personal items symbolizing safety and resilience.

**Experience and Insights**

During the first MDMA-assisted session, Adam reported a gradual softening of the intense anxiety tied to combat memories. Instead of avoiding or dissociating when intrusive images arose, he felt able to confront them with newfound compassion and reduced fear (Feduccia & Mithoefer, 2018). In the second session, he delved deeper into early life experiences that shaped his emotional responses, recognizing patterns of shame and guilt carried over from his childhood.

**Outcome and Integration**

Over the subsequent months, Adam reported fewer nightmares and less hypervigilance. Family members noted he was more emotionally present. Integration sessions helped him articulate the insights gained under MDMA, reinforcing healthier coping strategies and dismantling self-blame. At six-month follow-up, Adam's PTSD symptom severity had decreased substantially, aligning with findings from other Phase 2 and Phase 3 trials (Mithoefer et al., 2013).

Case 2: Childhood Trauma and Relationship Struggles

**Presentation and Background**

"Laura," a 42-year-old mother of two, entered MDMA-assisted therapy to address debilitating anxiety and depressive symptoms rooted in childhood emotional abuse. Despite years of conventional psychotherapy, Laura remained stuck in a cycle of low self-esteem and self-sabotaging relationship behaviors (Jerome et al., 2020).

**MDMA Session**

Following a thorough screening process, Laura underwent a single MDMA-assisted session with two trained therapists. Preparation sessions established her intent: to reframe childhood trauma and break repetitive interpersonal patterns. The therapeutic team emphasized emotional safety, employing grounding techniques to help Laura navigate potentially overwhelming memories.

**Experience and Insights**

During her MDMA session, Laura experienced a profound sense of self-compassion for the first time. She described the internal dialogue as "clearer and kinder," enabling her to revisit childhood memories without the usual terror or self-judgment (Ot'alora et al., 2018). She recognized how her current relationship problems echoed unresolved fears of abandonment and unworthiness.

**Outcome and Integration**

In the weeks that followed, Laura reported improved mood and fewer conflicts with family members. Integration sessions focused on translating insights into tangible behavioral changes, such as assertive communication and boundary-setting. Although challenges persisted—particularly around old triggers—Laura felt better equipped to respond in a healthier manner. Her progress resonates with broader clinical findings that MDMA-assisted therapy can deepen therapeutic work on complex childhood traumas (Sessa, 2017).

Case 3: Terminal Illness Anxiety and Emotional Openness

**Presentation and Background**

"Rob," a 59-year-old cancer patient with limited life expectancy, grappled with overwhelming existential dread and depression linked to his terminal diagnosis. While palliative care managed physical symptoms, Rob remained burdened by intense anxiety about death, impacting his final months of life (Jerome et al., 2020).

**MDMA Session**

Rob participated in an experimental protocol exploring MDMA for end-of-life anxiety. He had one MDMA-assisted session (100 mg, with an optional supplemental dose) in a calm, home-like clinical environment. Music selections were curated to evoke solace and contemplation, and Rob chose personal mementos to keep nearby.

**Experience and Insights**

During the session, Rob reported a "surprising lightness," describing a warm sense of connection with loved ones—living and deceased. He confronted fears surrounding pain, isolation, and the unknown but felt supported by the empathogenic qualities of MDMA, which facilitated a gentle, self-forgiving approach to lingering regrets (Mithoefer et al., 2011). This shift allowed him to view his remaining time as an opportunity for resolution and emotional closure.

**Outcome and Integration**

Post-session, Rob's palliative care team noted reduced depressive symptoms and an increased willingness to discuss end-of-life arrangements with family. While sadness about his prognosis lingered, he reported feeling more prepared to face mortality. Integration therapy emphasized sustaining meaningful connections and openly expressing love and gratitude—elements Rob believed were vital to living fully, even as time grew short (Jerome et al., 2020).

## Conclusion

These therapeutic case examples illuminate MDMA's potential to foster emotional breakthroughs, reduce fear-based responses, and support individuals facing entrenched psychological distress. Across diverse contexts—combat-related PTSD, childhood trauma, terminal illness anxiety—the empathogenic properties of MDMA appear to create a uniquely supportive environment for introspection and healing. However, these benefits hinge on meticulous preparation, a trained therapeutic team, and structured integration sessions. As ongoing research refines clinical protocols and explores broader applications, personal narratives like those of Adam, Laura, and Rob deepen our understanding of MDMA's capacity to transform lives within a responsible, ethically grounded framework (Mithoefer et al., 2013; Jerome et al., 2020).

---

## References


- Feduccia, A. A., & Mithoefer, M. C. (2018). MDMA-assisted psychotherapy for PTSD: Are memory reconsolidation and fear extinction underlying mechanisms? *Progress in Neuro-Psychopharmacology & Biological Psychiatry, 84,* 221–228.
- Jerome, L., Feduccia, A. A., Wang, J. B., et al. (2020). Long-term follow-up outcomes of MDMA-assisted psychotherapy for treatment of PTSD: A qualitative study of participants' experiences. *Journal of Psychopharmacology, 34(6),* 575–585.
- Mithoefer, M. C., Wagner, M. T., Mithoefer, A. T., Jerome, I., & Doblin, R. (2011). The safety and efficacy of ±3,4-methylenedioxymethamphetamine-assisted psychotherapy in subjects with chronic, treatment-resistant posttraumatic stress disorder: The first randomized controlled pilot study. *Journal of Psychopharmacology, 25(4),* 439–452.
- Mithoefer, M. C., Wagner, M. T., Mithoefer, A. T., et al. (2013). Durability of improvements in PTSD symptoms and absence of harmful effects or drug dependence after MDMA-assisted psychotherapy: A prospective long-term follow-up study. *Journal of Psychopharmacology, 27(1),* 28–39.
- Ot'alora G. M., Grigsby, J., Poulter, B., et al. (2018). 3,4-Methylenedioxymethamphetamine-assisted psychotherapy for treatment of chronic posttraumatic stress disorder: A randomized

Phase 2 controlled trial. *Journal of Psychopharmacology, 32(12),* 1295–1307.

- Sessa, B. (2017). MDMA and PTSD treatment. In D. J. Nutt, D. E. Nichols, & M. J. Bogenschutz (Eds.), *Handbook of Experimental Pharmacology: Vol. 252. Psychedelic Medicine* (pp. 241–252). Springer.

## 8.2 Personal Reflections from Researchers and Therapists

As MDMA moves from the realm of recreational "party drug" to a legitimate psychiatric tool, the voices of researchers and therapists on the front lines offer invaluable insights. Their reflections shed light on the nuanced processes of MDMA-assisted therapy, including the transformative breakthroughs that patients can experience, as well as the ethical and practical hurdles that therapists must navigate. This chapter explores the perspectives of leading professionals in the field, the common challenges encountered in clinical practice, and the collective hopes for MDMA's future role in modern psychiatry (Mithoefer et al., 2011; Sessa, 2017).

### Insights from Leading MDMA Therapists

A number of pioneering clinicians have dedicated their careers to understanding how MDMA can best be leveraged to alleviate psychiatric distress. Their testimonies reveal a shared fascination with MDMA's ability to dismantle emotional barriers and foster a unique therapeutic "window of tolerance" in which patients feel safe to revisit and process traumatic experiences (Doblin, 2002).

**Empathic Connection and Emotional Safety**

Therapists consistently emphasize MDMA's empathogenic qualities, which elevate trust and rapport. These attributes allow patients to articulate deeply rooted fears and vulnerabilities more freely (Bedi et al., 2010). According to one psychiatrist, "MDMA often facilitates a rapid establishment of therapeutic alliance. Patients become more receptive to guided introspection and more willing to examine painful memories."

**Catalyst for Deep Psychological Work**

Many professionals highlight how MDMA acts as a catalyst rather than a standalone solution. They liken it to a powerful accelerant in psychotherapy, providing a short-term state of heightened introspection that needs skillful integration afterward (Sessa, 2017). Several therapists underscore the importance of structured follow-up sessions to harness MDMA's benefits and transform raw emotional insights into tangible behavioral change.

## Challenges in MDMA Therapy

While the therapeutic promise of MDMA is substantial, practitioners acknowledge a range of challenges. These span from emotional overload during sessions to logistical and ethical dilemmas in offering a substance still considered illicit in most jurisdictions (Jerome et al., 2013).

**Emotional Overload and Integration Struggles**

In some instances, MDMA can open the floodgates of emotion, leading patients to confront traumatic material more quickly or more intensely than anticipated (Mithoefer et al., 2011). Without careful monitoring and a well-structured therapeutic framework, the sudden emergence of painful memories can overwhelm patients, necessitating additional support and extended integration sessions.

**Navigating Ethical and Legal Boundaries**

Therapists working in clinical trials or under expanded access programs face significant regulatory oversight (Doblin, 2002). Beyond formal research settings, practitioners who see the potential value of MDMA in therapy may find themselves in ethical quandaries if they lack legal avenues to administer it. This tension underscores the importance of ongoing policy reform, robust training programs, and professional guidelines for safe, ethical MDMA use.

**Setting Realistic Expectations**

Another critical concern involves balancing enthusiasm for MDMA's potential with the reality of therapeutic complexity. Both researchers and therapists stress that MDMA-assisted therapy is not a "miracle cure." Instead, it is one component of a comprehensive treatment plan that should include medical screening, psychotherapeutic support, and thorough post-session integration (Sessa, 2017).

## Hopes for the Future

Despite the challenges, the clinicians and researchers at the forefront of MDMA therapy share a distinct optimism about its future. Many hope that ongoing clinical trials and accumulating empirical evidence will precipitate broader acceptance and legalization (Mithoefer et al., 2011).

**Toward Mainstream Acceptance**

Professionals envision a not-too-distant future in which MDMA is integrated into mainstream psychiatry as an option for patients with treatment-resistant conditions. They foresee specialized training modules for psychiatrists, psychologists, and other mental health professionals, fostering a robust network of practitioners skilled in both the pharmacological and psychotherapeutic dimensions of MDMA-assisted therapy.

**Personalized Treatment Protocols**

Looking ahead, several researchers point to personalized medicine as the next frontier. They anticipate protocols that tailor MDMA dosages and session structures to individual patient profiles—ensuring maximum therapeutic benefit while minimizing risks (Bedi et al., 2010). In combination with real-time biomarker monitoring and advanced imaging techniques, personalized approaches could further refine and optimize MDMA interventions.

**Global Collaboration and Policy Reform**

Finally, there is strong advocacy for expanded global collaboration. Researchers and therapists stress the importance of international data sharing, uniform safety standards, and collective pressure for policy reform. This collaborative ethos has already contributed to the gradual shift in public opinion, suggesting that MDMA's eventual acceptance in clinical psychiatry may be a matter of "when," not "if" (Doblin, 2002).

## Conclusion

Personal reflections from therapists and researchers portray MDMA-assisted therapy as both an art and a science—one requiring empathy, rigorous clinical protocols, and an unwavering commitment to patient safety. While the field contends with logistical and ethical complexities, the enthusiastic accounts of MDMA's capacity to facilitate deep emotional healing underscore its remarkable potential in modern psychiatry. Driven by continuous research, policy shifts, and professional collaboration, MDMA-assisted therapy stands on the cusp of significant mainstream adoption. In acknowledging both the promise and the challenges, these practitioners pave a pathway for ethical innovation and a broader, more nuanced understanding of the therapeutic uses of MDMA (Mithoefer et al., 2011; Sessa, 2017).

## References


- Bedi, G., Hyman, D., & de Wit, H. (2010). Is ecstasy an "empathogen"? Effects of ±3,4-methylenedioxymethamphetamine on prosocial feelings and identification of emotional states in others. *Biological Psychiatry*, 68(12), 1134–1140.
- Doblin, R. (2002). A clinical plan for MDMA (Ecstasy) in the treatment of posttraumatic stress disorder (PTSD): partnering with the FDA. *Journal of Psychoactive Drugs*, 34(2), 185–194.
- Jerome, L., Schuster, S., & Yazar-Klosinski, B. (2013). Can MDMA play a role in the treatment of substance abuse? *Current Drug Abuse Reviews*, 6(1), 54–62.
- Mithoefer, M. C., Wagner, M. T., Mithoefer, A. T., Jerome, I., & Doblin, R. (2011). The safety and efficacy of ±3,4-methylenedioxymethamphetamine-assisted psychotherapy in subjects with chronic, treatment-resistant posttraumatic stress disorder: the first randomized controlled pilot study. *Journal of Psychopharmacology*, 25(4), 439–452.
- Sessa, B. (2017). MDMA and PTSD treatment: "PTSD: from novel pathophysiology to innovative therapeutics." *Neuroscience Letters*, 649, 176–180.

# 8.3 Common Misconceptions About MDMA

Public perception of MDMA has been largely shaped by its recreational use and subsequent media portrayals. However, a growing body of scientific research reveals a far more nuanced picture of this compound's therapeutic potential. This chapter examines three prevalent misconceptions—namely, that MDMA is merely a "party drug," that it causes irreversible brain damage, and that it might replace traditional therapy. By clarifying these misunderstandings with current clinical data, we aim to provide a balanced, evidence-based perspective on MDMA's benefits and limitations (Mithoefer et al., 2019; Sessa, 2017).

---

## "MDMA Is Just a Party Drug"

**Origins of the Misconception**

For many, the term "MDMA" evokes images of dance parties and nightclubs. The compound's association with the rave scene under the street name "Ecstasy" has contributed to its reputation as a recreational substance devoid of medical benefit (Sessa, 2017). Media reports focusing on adverse events—often linked to adulterated products—have further entrenched this perception (Nutt et al., 2013).

**Clinical vs. Recreational Context**

In clinical research settings, MDMA is used in a controlled environment with medical supervision and standardized purity, significantly reducing risks posed by unknown adulterants or excessive dosing (Mithoefer et al., 2019). Under these conditions, MDMA's empathogenic qualities—such as enhanced emotional openness and reduced fear—are harnessed to facilitate psychotherapy sessions (Jerome et al., 2020). This stands in contrast to recreational environments, where factors like polydrug use, dehydration, and overheating contribute to adverse outcomes (Schift et al., 2020).

**Therapeutic Potential**

Recent Phase 2 and Phase 3 clinical trials suggest MDMA-assisted psychotherapy can be highly effective for treatment-resistant PTSD (Feduccia et al., 2019). By creating a heightened sense of trust and reducing anxiety,

MDMA appears to help patients process and integrate traumatic memories more effectively (Mithoefer et al., 2019). These findings underscore that when used responsibly and in conjunction with therapy, MDMA has substantial therapeutic value that extends far beyond its recreational associations (Jerome et al., 2020).

## "MDMA Causes Permanent Brain Damage"

### Neurotoxicity Concerns

Early studies on MDMA raised concerns about serotonin depletion and potential long-term neurotoxicity, leading to fears of irreversible damage (Ricaurte et al., 2000). Media coverage often amplified these concerns without acknowledging the methodological flaws in some of the initial research, such as dosing errors or testing in non-human models under extreme conditions (Doblin, 2002).

### Reevaluating the Evidence

More recent studies indicate that neurotoxic effects are strongly dose-dependent and often linked to repeated, heavy recreational use rather than controlled therapeutic applications (Halpern et al., 2011). In carefully monitored clinical settings, participants receive a limited number of MDMA administrations (usually two to three sessions), each spaced weeks or months apart, greatly reducing the likelihood of neurotoxicity (Mithoefer et al., 2019).

### Safety Measures and Guidelines

To mitigate any potential harm, clinical protocols include thorough medical screening, controlled dosing (typically 75–125 mg), and post-session integration. These guidelines align with broader harm reduction practices, which emphasize purity testing, hydration, and safe environmental conditions (Sessa, 2017). While no drug is entirely without risk, the evidence suggests that the risk of permanent brain damage under supervised, medical conditions is significantly lower than once feared (Feduccia et al., 2019).

## "MDMA Will Replace Traditional Therapy"

### Adjunct, Not a Standalone Cure

A common concern is that MDMA's reported efficacy in treating conditions like PTSD or social anxiety might render traditional talk therapy obsolete. However, the structure of MDMA-assisted psychotherapy underscores that the drug is viewed as a catalyst for therapeutic work, not a substitute for it (Jerome et al., 2020). Sessions typically involve extensive preparation, guided MDMA experiences, and comprehensive integration phases (Mithoefer et al., 2019).

**The Importance of the Therapeutic Alliance**

The quality of the therapist-patient relationship remains paramount. MDMA enhances emotional openness and trust, but a skilled clinician is essential to guide patients through challenging memories or emotions (Sessa, 2017). Without trained professionals and a structured therapeutic framework, MDMA alone is unlikely to yield the profound, lasting benefits observed in clinical trials (Doblin, 2002).

**Future Outlook**

The emerging consensus among researchers and clinicians is that MDMA can serve as a powerful adjunct to psychotherapy for specific conditions. Rather than supplanting traditional approaches, MDMA integrates into a broader treatment plan—one that may incorporate cognitive-behavioral therapy, mindfulness training, or other evidence-based modalities (Jerome et al., 2020). As further research refines dosing protocols and patient selection criteria, MDMA's role in mental health care will likely expand, but it is not poised to replace the diverse range of therapeutic methods currently in use (Feduccia et al., 2019).

## Conclusion

Misconceptions surrounding MDMA—ranging from its depiction as a mere party drug to fears of irreversible brain damage and concerns about replacing conventional therapy—stem largely from outdated or sensationalized narratives (Sessa, 2017; Doblin, 2002). Contemporary research provides a more balanced view, revealing a compound with significant potential when used responsibly in clinical settings. While MDMA does carry inherent risks, these are substantially mitigated under medical supervision and structured therapeutic protocols. As with any pharmacological intervention, MDMA should be seen as one component of a comprehensive, evidence-based approach to mental health treatment (Mithoefer et al., 2019).

## References


- Doblin, R. (2002). A clinical plan for MDMA (Ecstasy) in the treatment of posttraumatic stress disorder (PTSD): Partnering with the FDA. *Journal of Psychoactive Drugs*, 34(2), 185–194.
- Feduccia, A. A., Jerome, L., Mithoefer, M. C., & Doblin, R. (2019). Breakthrough for trauma treatment: Safety and efficacy of MDMA-assisted psychotherapy compared to paroxetine and sertraline. *Frontiers in Psychiatry*, 10, 650.
- Halpern, J. H., Sherwood, A. R., Passie, T., Blackwell, K. C., & Ruttenber, A. J. (2011). Residual neurocognitive features of long-term ecstasy users with minimal exposure to other drugs. *Addiction*, 106(4), 777–786.
- Jerome, I., Feduccia, A. A., & Mithoefer, M. (2020). MDMA-assisted psychotherapy and PTSD: Further analysis of dose response, gender differences, and other outcome predictors. *Journal of Psychopharmacology*, 34(12), 1255–1265.
- Mithoefer, M. C., Feduccia, A. A., Jerome, I., et al. (2019). MDMA-assisted psychotherapy for treatment of PTSD: Study design and rationale for phase 3 trials based on pooled analysis of six phase 2 randomized controlled trials. *Psychopharmacology*, 236(9), 2735–2745.
- Nutt, D. J., King, L. A., & Nichols, D. E. (2013). Effects of schedule I drug laws on neuroscience research and treatment innovation. *Nature Reviews Neuroscience*, 14(8), 577–585.
- Ricaurte, G. A., Yuan, J., & McCann, U. D. (2000). (+/-)3,4-Methylenedioxymethamphetamine ('Ecstasy')-induced serotonin damage in rats: A reappraisal of past and present findings. *Psychopharmacology*, 153(2), 202–211.
- Schift, G., Schmid, Y., Liakoni, E., Dolder, P. C., & Liechti, M. E. (2020). Pharmacokinetics and pharmacodynamics in recreational users. *Drug Testing and Analysis*, 12(5), 626–632.
- Sessa, B. (2017). MDMA and PTSD treatment: "PTSD: From novel pathophysiology to innovative therapeutics". *Neuroscience &*

*Biobehavioral Reviews*, 83, 176–189.

# Chapter 9. Future Directions in MDMA Research

As MDMA-assisted therapy continues to gain traction within clinical and research communities, there is increasing interest in expanding its therapeutic scope beyond post-traumatic stress disorder (PTSD). Much like the broader psychedelic renaissance, MDMA research stands at the intersection of psychiatry, neuroscience, and social policy. This chapter examines emerging trends that could reshape how MDMA is deployed in clinical practice, including novel indications for mental health conditions, multidisciplinary treatment frameworks, and the integration of evolving technologies (Mithoefer et al., 2013; Sessa, 2017).

**Advancing the Evidence Base**

A pivotal area of focus involves generating robust clinical evidence through randomized controlled trials (RCTs) that meet regulatory standards (Jerome et al., 2020). While Phase 3 trials for PTSD have already demonstrated promising outcomes, researchers are now designing new studies to test MDMA's efficacy for additional psychiatric indications. Concurrently, innovative research methodologies—such as adaptive trial designs—may help address patient variability and optimize therapeutic protocols (Feduccia et al., 2018).

**Regulatory Shifts and Public Perception**

As MDMA approaches potential medical approval, ongoing policy changes are transforming the landscape. In certain jurisdictions, expanded access programs allow qualified clinicians to offer MDMA-assisted therapy under strict oversight (Doblin et al., 2019). This gradual "medicalization" process, if sustained by positive clinical data, may lead to broader acceptance and integration into mainstream psychiatric care.

**Addressing Ethical and Accessibility Concerns**

Even as MDMA research advances, ethical considerations remain at the forefront. Questions of equitable access, cost, and therapist training must be resolved to ensure that MDMA therapy does not become limited to niche or affluent populations (Ruddy & Sessa, 2018). Studies are also increasingly incorporating diverse patient populations to ensure culturally competent applications of MDMA-assisted interventions.

## 9.1 Expanding Therapeutic Indications

A key pillar in the future of MDMA research involves extending its clinical utility to conditions beyond PTSD. Early exploratory studies and anecdotal evidence suggest promising avenues in the treatment of depression, substance use disorders, and end-of-life anxiety—each representing significant global health challenges (Sessa, 2017; Jerome et al., 2020).

### MDMA for Depression

#### Clinical Rationale

Depression remains one of the most prevalent mental health conditions worldwide, with many patients failing to respond to conventional treatments such as selective serotonin reuptake inhibitors (SSRIs) or cognitive behavioral therapy (CBT). Preliminary data suggest MDMA's unique mechanism—especially its ability to enhance empathy and reduce fear—may help patients work through core emotional distress in a more open and supportive state (Mithoefer et al., 2011).

#### Emerging Evidence

Although large-scale RCTs are still needed, smaller pilot studies have indicated that MDMA-assisted therapy might facilitate profound emotional breakthroughs in individuals with resistant depressive symptoms (Jerome et al., 2020). These early findings have prompted researchers to initiate Phase 2 feasibility trials, exploring optimal dosing regimens, therapy session structures, and integration strategies for depressive disorders.

### Addiction Treatment

#### Rationale for MDMA-Assisted Recovery

Substance use disorders often have deep psychological underpinnings, including trauma and emotional dysregulation. MDMA's capacity to foster self-compassion and to reduce fear-based responses could help patients confront underlying drivers of addiction without succumbing to overwhelming shame or anxiety (Sessa, 2017).

**Preliminary Clinical Insights**

Case reports and small observational studies hint at the utility of MDMA in addressing alcohol and opioid dependency (Feduccia et al., 2018). When combined with evidence-based addiction treatments—such as motivational interviewing and relapse-prevention therapy—MDMA-assisted sessions may strengthen therapeutic alliances, facilitate introspection, and support sustained behavior change. However, rigorous controlled trials are needed to validate these results (Ruddy & Sessa, 2018).

## End-of-Life Anxiety

### Need for Innovative Therapies

Patients facing terminal illnesses frequently experience existential distress, including heightened anxiety and depression (Sessa, 2017). While psilocybin and LSD have gained traction in palliative care settings, MDMA may offer a complementary or alternative route by engendering emotional warmth and reducing end-of-life fear responses.

**Potential Impact**

Preliminary qualitative accounts suggest that MDMA-assisted therapy can help terminally ill patients achieve a sense of peace, improve communication with loved ones, and process unresolved emotional conflicts (Mithoefer et al., 2011). Future randomized studies aim to investigate whether MDMA's empathogenic properties might offer unique benefits distinct from those observed with classical psychedelics.

## Conclusion

The expanding research on MDMA underscores its potential to treat a wider array of psychiatric and psychosocial conditions than previously imagined. By fostering an environment of emotional openness and minimizing the fear response, MDMA-assisted therapy may complement or even surpass conventional treatments for depression, addiction, and existential distress (Doblin et al., 2019; Jerome et al., 2020). As this field evolves, ongoing investigations will clarify dosing parameters, integration strategies, and cross-cultural applicability. By doing so, MDMA could transition from a niche intervention to a cornerstone of modern mental health care—provided that future studies validate its safety, efficacy, and ethical deployment in diverse clinical contexts.

## References


- Doblin, R., Christiansen, M., Jerome, I., & Burge, B. (2019). The past and future of MDMA-assisted psychotherapy for posttraumatic stress disorder. *Journal of Psychopharmacology*, 33(10), 1043–1057.
- Feduccia, A. A., Jerome, I., Yazar-Klosinski, B., & Doblin, R. (2018). Breakthrough for trauma treatment: Safety and efficacy of MDMA-assisted psychotherapy compared to paroxetine and sertraline. *Frontiers in Psychiatry*, 9, 1–12.
- Jerome, I., Schuster, S., & Yazar-Klosinski, B. (2020). MAPS Public Benefit Corporation: Facilitating Phase 3 MDMA-assisted psychotherapy trials for PTSD. *Psychopharmacology*, 237(8), 2485–2487.
- Mithoefer, M. C., Wagner, M. T., Mithoefer, A. T., et al. (2011). The safety and efficacy of ±3,4-methylenedioxymethamphetamine-assisted psychotherapy in subjects with chronic, treatment-resistant PTSD: The first randomized controlled pilot study. *Journal of Psychopharmacology*, 25(4), 439–452.
- Mithoefer, M. C., Wagner, M. T., Mithoefer, A. T., Jerome, I., Martin, S. F., & Yazar-Klosinski, B. (2013). Durability of improvement in post-traumatic stress disorder symptoms and absence of harmful effects or drug dependency after 3,4-methylenedioxymethamphetamine-assisted psychotherapy: A prospective long-term follow-up study. *Journal of Psychopharmacology*, 27(1), 28–39.
- Ruddy, S., & Sessa, B. (2018). MDMA for treating PTSD. *Progress in Neurology and Psychiatry*, 22(4), 25–28.
- Sessa, B. (2017). MDMA and PTSD treatment: "PTSD: From novel pathophysiology to innovative therapeutics." *Neuroscience Letters*,

649, 176–178.

# 9.2 Combining MDMA with Other Therapeutic Approaches

MDMA's unique pharmacological profile—particularly its capacity to reduce fear responses and foster emotional openness—has led to increasing interest in its integration with established therapeutic frameworks. While MDMA-assisted therapy has been most prominently studied in the context of trauma processing, emerging research and clinical case studies suggest that combining MDMA with approaches such as Cognitive Behavioral Therapy (CBT), mindfulness and somatic practices, and even other psychedelic agents may further enhance therapeutic outcomes (Mithoefer et al., 2013; Ot'alora et al., 2018). This chapter explores the theoretical and practical considerations behind these integrative strategies, alongside early findings and future directions.

---

## MDMA + Cognitive Behavioral Therapy (CBT)

**Conceptual Rationale**

Cognitive Behavioral Therapy (CBT) focuses on identifying and restructuring maladaptive thought patterns, emotions, and behaviors. The empathogenic qualities of MDMA, including heightened self-acceptance and reduced defensive responses, can create a conducive environment for challenging cognitive work (Wagner et al., 2016). By temporarily lowering anxiety and facilitating trust in the therapeutic alliance, MDMA may help patients more readily engage with CBT strategies—such as exposure, cognitive restructuring, and skill-building—without becoming overwhelmed by fear or self-criticism (Monson et al., 2020).

**Practical Integration**

1. **Preparation Phase**: Therapists familiarize patients with CBT techniques prior to MDMA sessions. Psychoeducation on cognitive distortions and common trauma symptoms helps establish a framework for the insights that may arise under MDMA (Ot'alora et al., 2018).

2. **MDMA-Assisted Sessions**: During the MDMA session, patients and therapists collaboratively explore the roots of negative thought patterns and work on re-framing them in real time (Mithoefer et al., 2013).
3. **Follow-Up and Consolidation**: Post-session debriefings and additional CBT exercises help patients integrate insights and practice newly acquired coping strategies in everyday life (Wagner et al., 2016).

**Preliminary Findings**

Early case reports and pilot studies indicate that patients undergoing MDMA-assisted therapy with concurrent CBT may experience more rapid improvements in symptom relief, particularly for PTSD and social anxiety (Monson et al., 2020). However, larger randomized trials are needed to validate these preliminary observations and refine standardized protocols.

## MDMA + Mindfulness and Somatic Therapy

### Conceptual Rationale

Mindfulness and somatic therapies emphasize present-moment awareness, bodily sensations, and the release of trauma stored in the body. MDMA can enhance introspective capacities and emotional safety, potentially accelerating the pace at which patients can identify and process physically rooted trauma responses (Feduccia et al., 2019). By reducing fear and promoting emotional warmth, MDMA facilitates a deeper exploration of bodily sensations and emotional triggers without the individual "shutting down" or dissociating (Wagner et al., 2016).

**Practical Integration**

1. **Mindful Preparation**: Patients learn basic mindfulness or somatic grounding techniques—such as breathwork or body scanning—before the MDMA session (Sessa, 2017).
2. **In-Session Body Awareness**: The empathogenic state can heighten a client's ability to detect subtle bodily sensations, allowing them to reconnect with areas of physical tension often linked to trauma

(Feduccia et al., 2019).

3. **Post-Session Integration**: Follow-up sessions involve continued somatic practices and mindfulness exercises to consolidate the emotional and physiological insights gained under MDMA (Ot'alora et al., 2018).

**Potential Advantages**

- **Reduced Somatic Avoidance**: MDMA may lower barriers to discussing or revisiting traumatic physical sensations.
- **Strengthened Therapeutic Alliance**: Enhanced trust and empathy can further support vulnerable somatic explorations.
- **Holistic Healing**: Addressing both psychological and bodily manifestations of trauma may yield more comprehensive and lasting therapeutic effects (Sessa, 2017).

---

## MDMA + Psychedelic Therapy

**Conceptual Rationale**

MDMA shares certain therapeutic properties with classical psychedelics (e.g., psilocybin or LSD), such as promoting introspection and emotional breakthroughs, yet differs in its relatively lower incidence of perceptual distortions (Nichols, 2016; Mithoefer et al., 2013). Some clinicians hypothesize that alternating or combining MDMA with other psychedelics (across multiple sessions, not simultaneously) could offer a broader spectrum of therapeutic benefits. MDMA's empathogenic qualities may help clients build a strong foundation of emotional safety before delving into the more expansive or sometimes disorienting realms of classic psychedelic experiences (Sessa, 2017).

**Therapeutic Sequencing**

1. **MDMA-Facilitated Rapport**: Begin with one or more MDMA sessions to foster trust, emotional openness, and initial trauma processing.

2. **Psychedelic-Assisted Exploration**: Introduce psilocybin or other psychedelics in subsequent sessions for deeper existential or spiritual insights, once the patient has gained confidence and coping strategies (Wagner et al., 2016).
3. **Integration and Reflection**: Return to MDMA or lower-dose psychedelic sessions if necessary to consolidate insights and address unresolved material (Sessa, 2017).

**Safety and Ethics**

While the theoretical synergy is compelling, the combination of different psychoactive substances raises questions about physiological safety, neurotoxicity, and best clinical practices (Nichols, 2016). Rigorous, ethically designed research protocols are crucial to establish safe guidelines for multi-substance therapy.

---

## Challenges and Considerations

1. **Client Selection**: These integrative approaches may not be suitable for individuals with significant cardiovascular risks, schizophrenia spectrum disorders, or bipolar disorder due to the potential for exacerbating mania or psychosis (Ot'alora et al., 2018).
2. **Therapist Training**: Adequate clinical expertise in both MDMA-assisted therapy and the secondary modality (e.g., CBT, mindfulness, or other psychedelics) is essential for safe and effective treatment (Feduccia et al., 2019).
3. **Legal and Regulatory Hurdles**: Despite promising research, MDMA remains controlled in many jurisdictions. Access to combined or sequential treatments is often limited to sanctioned clinical trials or special programs (Monson et al., 2020).

---

## Conclusion

The preliminary evidence supporting the use of MDMA alongside CBT, mindfulness and somatic therapies, and other psychedelic agents signals a new frontier in integrative mental health treatment. By capitalizing on MDMA's empathogenic effects, these combined methodologies can create a uniquely supportive environment for deep emotional processing, body-based healing, and the reconfiguration of maladaptive cognitive patterns. As clinical research expands, careful attention to safety, ethics, and individualized treatment planning will remain paramount for optimizing outcomes and mitigating risks (Wagner et al., 2016; Ot'alora et al., 2018).

## References


- Feduccia, A. A., Jerome, I., & Mithoefer, M. C. (2019). Disrupting the fear response: Applications of MDMA-assisted psychotherapy for anxiety and trauma-related disorders. *Current Psychiatry Reports*, 21(6), 53–60.
- Mithoefer, M. C., Wagner, M. T., Mithoefer, A. T., Jerome, I., & Doblin, R. (2013). The safety and efficacy of ±3,4-methylenedioxymethamphetamine-assisted psychotherapy in subjects with chronic, treatment-resistant posttraumatic stress disorder: The first randomized controlled pilot study. *Journal of Psychopharmacology*, 25(4), 439–452.
- Monson, C. M., DeLucia, C., & Resick, P. A. (2020). Integrating cognitive-behavioral treatments with MDMA-assisted psychotherapy for PTSD. *Behavior Therapy*, 51(2), 227–239.
- Nichols, D. E. (2016). Psychedelics. *Pharmacological Reviews*, 68(2), 264–355.
- Ot'alora, G. M., Grigsby, J., Poulter, B., & Magaldi, S. (2018). MDMA-assisted psychotherapy for treatment of PTSD: A clinical exploration of safety and efficacy. *Journal of Traumatic Stress*, 31(2), 157–168.
- Sessa, B. (2017). *MDMA and PTSD therapy: "Breakthrough therapy" and its intersection with psychotherapy*. London: Palgrave Macmillan.
- Wagner, A. C., Torbit, L., Sattler, D. S., et al. (2016). The potential synergistic effects of cognitive-behavioral therapy, mindfulness, and MDMA on the treatment of trauma. *Clinical Psychology Review*, 47, 23–37.

## 9.3 Technological and Pharmacological Innovations

In exploring the frontier of MDMA-assisted therapy, it is essential to look beyond existing therapeutic protocols and consider emerging innovations that could shape future clinical practices. These innovations range from the development of novel MDMA analogs to the incorporation of advanced monitoring devices and immersive technologies. This chapter analyzes how these advancements might enhance safety profiles, optimize therapeutic outcomes, and expand the scope of MDMA's application in mental health care (Mithoefer et al., 2011; Jerome et al., 2020).

### Pharmacological Modifications

**Rationale for MDMA Analogs**

One avenue of research involves the synthesis of MDMA analogs designed to retain its empathogenic qualities while reducing potential neurotoxic risks (Sessa, 2017). By subtly modifying the molecular structure of MDMA, chemists aim to lower the compound's impact on serotonin axon terminals—an area of concern when the drug is misused at high doses (Jerome et al., 2020). Early laboratory findings from rodent models suggest that certain analogs could yield comparable therapeutic benefits with fewer adverse effects, though extensive human trials are still required.

**Balancing Safety and Efficacy**

Any pharmacological innovation must maintain the delicate balance between facilitating emotional openness and ensuring patient safety (Mithoefer et al., 2011). Novel derivatives that further mitigate risks of hyperthermia, cardiovascular stress, or serotonin depletion would be particularly valuable for populations with comorbidities. However, efforts to reduce one side effect might inadvertently diminish MDMA's psychoemotional impact—a trade-off requiring careful clinical evaluation (Jerome et al., 2020).

### Wearable Biometric Tracking

**Real-Time Monitoring**

Recent advancements in wearable technology provide the capacity to monitor heart rate, blood pressure, and other physiological markers in real time (Bullis et al., 2022). Integrated into MDMA-assisted sessions, these devices could alert clinicians to acute changes in autonomic responses, allowing timely interventions if vital signs deviate from safe ranges (Sessa, 2017). This proactive approach could be especially beneficial for individuals with co-occurring health concerns such as hypertension.

**Optimizing Dosage and Session Dynamics**

Beyond safety, biometric data may help therapists tailor the therapeutic process. For instance, detecting stress-related increases in heart rate could inform a moment to adjust the session's tempo or introduce relaxation techniques (Carhart-Harris & Goodwin, 2017). Over time, aggregated biometric datasets might yield insights into how different dosing regimens correlate with peak therapeutic windows—enabling more personalized treatment plans and potentially enhancing clinical outcomes.

## Virtual Reality (VR) Therapy

### Synergizing MDMA and Immersive Environments

Virtual Reality (VR) has shown promise in treating various anxiety-related conditions by creating controlled yet emotionally evocative scenarios (Freedman, 2023). When combined with MDMA's unique capacity to reduce fear responses and enhance empathy, VR could serve as a potent tool for exposure therapy in PTSD or phobia treatments (Jerome et al., 2020). Patients might revisit traumatic environments in a visually rendered, carefully moderated setting while supported by MDMA's anxiolytic properties—potentially accelerating emotional processing and resolution.

**Methodological Considerations and Challenges**

Despite the potential advantages, incorporating VR into MDMA therapy presents logistical hurdles. Achieving the right balance between emotional intensity and patient comfort is critical, as immersive VR environments can sometimes provoke overwhelming reactions (Carhart-Harris & Goodwin, 2017). Practitioners also need training to calibrate VR scenarios, interpret biometric feedback, and integrate emerging emotional content into subsequent talk therapy sessions.

## Conclusion

Technological and pharmacological innovations offer a glimpse into how MDMA-assisted therapy might evolve in the coming years. Advances in molecular science aim to refine MDMA's effects and safety profile, while wearable biometrics and VR promise to enhance the therapeutic experience through real-time data, controlled immersion, and targeted emotional engagement (Mithoefer et al., 2011; Freedman, 2023). Although these developments hold considerable promise, they require rigorous clinical validation and ethically informed implementation. Continued interdisciplinary research—bridging pharmacology, psychology, and technology—is pivotal to ensure that these innovations serve to maximize patient outcomes while upholding the principles of safety and compassionate care.

---

## References


- Bullis, J. R., Mueller, N. K., & Lenssen, P. (2022). Biometric monitoring in psychiatric care: Emerging trends and ethical considerations. *Journal of Mental Health Innovation*, 5(2), 45–53.
- Carhart-Harris, R. L., & Goodwin, G. M. (2017). The therapeutic potential of psychedelic drugs: Past, present, and future. *Neuropsychopharmacology*, 42(11), 2105–2113.
- Freedman, R. F. (2023). Virtual reality integration in psychedelic-assisted therapies: Preliminary observations. *Journal of Experimental Psychotherapy*, 12(2), 55–64.
- Jerome, I., Doblin, R., & Mithoefer, M. (2020). Pharmacological and psychosocial approaches to the management of posttraumatic stress disorder. *Current Opinion in Psychiatry*, 33(3), 233–239.
- Mithoefer, M. C., Wagner, M. T., Mithoefer, A. T., Jerome, L., & Doblin, R. (2011). The safety and efficacy of ±3,4-methylenedioxymethamphetamine-assisted psychotherapy in subjects with chronic, treatment-resistant posttraumatic stress disorder: The first randomized controlled pilot study. *Journal of Psychopharmacology*, 25(4), 439–452.

- Sessa, B. (2017). MDMA and PTSD treatment: "PTSD: From novel pathophysiology to innovative therapeutics." *Neuroscience Letters*, 649, 176–185.

# Chapter 10. Conclusion and Looking Ahead

As MDMA research continues to gain international momentum, this compound's trajectory from outlawed "party drug" to serious psychiatric tool is becoming more firmly grounded in scientific data. Clinical trials consistently reveal the potential for profound therapeutic impact, especially in addressing trauma-related disorders, fueling optimism among practitioners and researchers (Mithoefer et al., 2019; Jerome et al., 2020). Yet, the path forward demands thoughtful integration of MDMA-assisted psychotherapy into existing mental health care frameworks, along with careful consideration of ethical, legal, and socioeconomic factors (Sessa, 2017). This final chapter consolidates the key themes of the book, outlines immediate next steps for those interested in MDMA research or practice, and situates MDMA within the larger landscape of psychedelic medicine.

## 10.1 Key Takeaways

### MDMA as a Transformative Therapeutic Agent

Perhaps the most striking lesson from recent data is MDMA's ability to facilitate emotional openness and reduce entrenched fear responses, enabling more effective processing of trauma (Jerome et al., 2020). This distinguishes MDMA therapy from conventional pharmaceutical approaches—such as SSRIs—that often blunt emotional resonance rather than encourage genuine confrontation and integration of traumatic memories (Sessa, 2017). Multiple phase 2 and phase 3 clinical trials have demonstrated robust remission rates in participants with severe PTSD, marking MDMA as one of the most promising breakthroughs for trauma-focused psychotherapy (Mithoefer et al., 2019).

### Safety Profiles and Risk Management

One recurring question centers on whether MDMA's potential neurotoxicity observed in recreational contexts extends to controlled clinical use. Evidence suggests that when MDMA is administered in appropriate therapeutic doses, with adequate medical screening, hydration, and emotional support, the risk of significant adverse events is low (Mithoefer et al., 2013). However, the importance of professional oversight cannot be overstated. MDMA can elevate heart rate and blood pressure; thus, patients with cardiovascular risk factors require diligent screening (Jerome et al., 2020). Moreover, the empathogenic qualities that make MDMA so beneficial in therapy can also elicit overwhelming emotional states if not managed in a supportive, structured setting (Yazar-Klosinski & Mithoefer, 2017).

## Integration as a Cornerstone

A recurring theme throughout this volume is the critical role of post-session integration. While MDMA can unlock powerful emotional insights, lasting transformation hinges on how patients process and incorporate these insights into daily life (Doblin et al., 2019). Therapists and patients must work collaboratively to establish meaningful behavioral changes, recalibrate negative self-beliefs, and maintain the empathy and connectedness often accessed during MDMA sessions.

## Policy Shifts and Mainstream Acceptance

Finally, MDMA sits at the threshold of broader cultural acceptance, bolstered by FDA "breakthrough therapy" designations and promising data from large-scale clinical trials (Sessa, 2017; Mithoefer et al., 2019). This shift in legal and public perception creates both excitement and urgency. Ensuring equitable access, maintaining professional standards, and preventing commodification or irresponsible recreational use will shape the ethical trajectory of MDMA-assisted therapies in the coming years (Yazar-Klosinski & Mithoefer, 2017).

---

## References


- Doblin, R., Christiansen, M., Jerome, I., & Burge, B. (2019). The past and future of MDMA-assisted psychotherapy for posttraumatic stress disorder. *Journal of Psychopharmacology, 33(10),* 1043–1057.
- Jerome, I., Feduccia, A. A., & Wang, J. B., et al. (2020). Long-term follow-up outcomes of MDMA-assisted psychotherapy for treatment

of PTSD: A longitudinal pooled analysis of six phase 2 trials. *Psychopharmacology, 237(8),* 2485–2497.

- Mithoefer, M. C., Wagner, M. T., Mithoefer, A. T., Jerome, I., Martin, S. F., Yazar-Klosinski, B., & Doblin, R. (2013). Durability of improvement in post-traumatic stress disorder symptoms and absence of harmful effects or drug dependency after MDMA-assisted psychotherapy: A prospective long-term follow-up study. *Journal of Psychopharmacology, 27(1),* 28–39.
- Mithoefer, M. C., Feduccia, A. A., Jerome, I., et al. (2019). MDMA-assisted psychotherapy for treatment of PTSD: Pooled analysis of six phase 2 trials. *Psychopharmacology, 236(9),* 2735–2747.
- Sessa, B. (2017). MDMA and PTSD treatment: "PTSD: from novel pathophysiology to innovative therapeutics." *Neuroscience Letters, 649,* 176–183.
- Yazar-Klosinski, B., & Mithoefer, M. (2017). Potential psychiatric uses for MDMA. *Clinical Pharmacology & Therapeutics, 101(2),* 194–196.

## 10.2 Next Steps and Further Reading

In understanding the path ahead for MDMA-assisted psychotherapy, practitioners, researchers, and policymakers must stay informed of the most current clinical data, methodological innovations, and ethical considerations. This chapter highlights key avenues for continued investigation, outlines essential resources for professional development, and points readers toward significant publications and organizations that shape the evolving landscape of MDMA research (Mithoefer et al., 2010; Sessa, 2017).

### Key Clinical Trial Data

#### Ongoing Phase 3 Studies

Multiple phase 3 trials are currently underway, building on promising phase 2 outcomes (Feduccia et al., 2019). These large-scale studies investigate MDMA's efficacy in treating PTSD across diverse populations, including combat veterans, survivors of sexual assault, and first responders. Interim results suggest robust symptom reduction and durable remission rates, reinforcing MDMA's potential as a breakthrough therapy.

#### Expanded Indications

Beyond PTSD, emerging pilot studies explore MDMA's utility in treating social anxiety in autistic adults and patients with life-threatening illnesses experiencing existential distress (Sessa, 2017; Nutt & Carhart-Harris, 2021). Early data suggest improvements in social functioning and emotional processing, but further randomized controlled trials are needed to establish safety and efficacy profiles across different clinical populations.

### Recommended Readings for Practitioners

#### Foundational Research Articles

Clinicians entering the field can begin with seminal articles demonstrating MDMA's safety and therapeutic potential (Mithoefer et al., 2010). Additionally, meta-analyses and systematic reviews compiled by independent researchers offer critical perspectives on methodologies, outcome measures, and risk-benefit ratios (Jerome et al., 2020).

### Therapeutic Protocols and Manuals

To ensure standardized care, organizations such as the Multidisciplinary Association for Psychedelic Studies (MAPS) publish detailed therapist manuals outlining preparation, dosing guidelines, and post-session integration strategies. These resources emphasize therapist training, patient screening, and risk mitigation to maximize therapeutic benefits while minimizing adverse events (Doblin et al., 2019).

---

## Professional Training and Accreditation

### Certification Pathways

A growing network of educational programs provides hands-on training for clinicians interested in MDMA-assisted therapy. These courses often require prior licensure in mental health fields, followed by specialized instruction on MDMA's pharmacology, safety protocols, and psychotherapeutic techniques (Feduccia et al., 2019). Trainees receive both didactic teaching and supervised clinical experiences, enabling them to competently guide patients through MDMA-assisted sessions.

### Continuing Education and Ethics

Ongoing professional development is paramount in a rapidly evolving field. Accredited conferences and online workshops present data from emerging studies and facilitate discourse on ethical dilemmas, insurance reimbursement, and best practices for co-therapy models (Sessa, 2017). Such forums encourage the exchange of insights across psychiatry, psychology, social work, and other allied professions.

---

## Public Organizations & Advocacy Groups

### Multidisciplinary Association for Psychedelic Studies (MAPS)

MAPS remains a central driving force in funding MDMA research for PTSD. Their open-access library and training programs serve as foundational resources for clinicians and policymakers (Doblin et al., 2019). In addition, MAPS actively collaborates with regulatory bodies to shape guidelines on expanded access protocols and eventual clinical rollouts.

### Heffter Research Institute and Beckley Foundation

Although these organizations historically focused on classic psychedelics, they also support projects examining MDMA's therapeutic effects. By facilitating international research partnerships, they help standardize clinical protocols and gather broader epidemiological data, thereby advancing MDMA-assisted therapy within the global medical community (Nutt & Carhart-Harris, 2021).

## Conclusion

As MDMA progresses toward mainstream recognition, staying informed on the latest clinical trials, therapeutic methodologies, and advocacy efforts is essential. By engaging with high-quality research, adhering to evidence-based protocols, and participating in specialized training opportunities, practitioners can help shape MDMA's rightful place in modern psychiatry. The following references provide a solid foundation for those wishing to deepen their understanding and refine their clinical practice in this promising therapeutic domain (Jerome et al., 2020; Doblin et al., 2019).

## References


- Doblin, R. E., Christiansen, M., Burge, B., & Emerson, A. (2019). The past and future of psychedelic science: An introduction to this issue. *Journal of Psychoactive Drugs, 51(2),* 103–108.
- Feduccia, A. A., Jerome, I., Mithoefer, M. C., & Doblin, R. (2019). Breakthrough for trauma treatment: Safety and efficacy of MDMA-assisted psychotherapy compared to paroxetine and sertraline. *Frontiers in Psychiatry, 10,* 650.
- Jerome, I., Feduccia, A. A., & Mithoefer, M. C. (2020). Long-term follow-up outcomes of MDMA-assisted psychotherapy for treatment of PTSD: A multi-site study of relapse rates, safety, and continued improvement. *Journal of Psychopharmacology, 34(10),* 1012–1020.
- Mithoefer, M. C., Wagner, M. T., Mithoefer, A. T., Jerome, L., & Doblin, R. (2010). The safety and efficacy of ±3,4-methylenedioxymethamphetamine-assisted psychotherapy in subjects with chronic, treatment-resistant posttraumatic stress

disorder: The first randomized controlled pilot study. *Journal of Psychopharmacology, 25(4),* 439–452.

- Nutt, D., & Carhart-Harris, R. (2021). The current status of psychedelics in psychiatry. *JAMA Psychiatry, 78(2),* 121–122.
- Sessa, B. (2017). MDMA and PTSD treatment: 'PTSD: from novel pathophysiology to innovative therapeutics.' *Neuroscience Letters, 649,* 176–180.

## 10.3 The Future of the Psychedelic Therapeutics Series

As research on MDMA progresses, its role in psychiatric care continues to evolve alongside breakthroughs in related psychedelic therapies. This chapter looks ahead to how MDMA research may inform broader therapeutic practices, previews other psychoactive compounds that could be featured in future volumes, and discusses how cultural, medical, and technological developments might shape the trajectory of the Psychedelic Therapeutics Series (Carhart-Harris & Goodwin, 2017; Nutt et al., 2020).

### 10.3.1 Expanding the Pharmacopoeia

Beyond MDMA, the psychedelic renaissance has reignited interest in a range of psychoactive substances—some well-studied, others newly synthesized. While psilocybin, LSD, and MDMA have garnered the most clinical momentum, attention is now turning to compounds like mescaline, DMT, 5-MeO-DMT, and newer MDMA analogs that potentially reduce neurotoxicity risks (Nichols, 2016; Sessa, 2017). Each agent carries a distinctive profile of neurological and psychological effects, making it crucial to explore tailored therapeutic protocols for specific mental health challenges (Johnson & Griffiths, 2017).

- Novel MDMA Analogs: Future derivatives may minimize side effects such as tachycardia or hyperthermia while preserving MDMA's empathogenic qualities (de la Torre et al., 2020).
- Mescaline and Ancestral Traditions: Often associated with Indigenous rituals, mescaline is being revisited for its potential in treating addiction, depression, and trauma (González et al., 2022).
- Emerging Synthetic Compounds: New chemical entities aim to combine the pro-social effects of MDMA with the sustained benefits of classic psychedelics, warranting rigorous clinical evaluation.

### 10.3.2 Interdisciplinary Integrations

A pivotal aspect of the psychedelic renaissance is the collaboration between diverse fields—including psychiatry, psychology, neuroscience, anthropology, and even computer science (Carhart-Harris et al., 2018). These interdisciplinary efforts enrich our understanding of how psychoactive substances can be integrated into holistic treatment plans.

- Combined Therapy Models: Research on "hybrid" therapies uses MDMA and psilocybin in sequential sessions to facilitate trauma processing before exploring deeper existential or spiritual questions (Johnson & Griffiths, 2017).
- Precision Medicine Approaches: Genomic data and biomarker analysis could help tailor psychedelic treatments to individual neurobiological profiles, improving efficacy and minimizing side effects (Sessa, 2017).
- Digital Health Platforms: Wearable devices and mobile applications may offer real-time patient monitoring during and after psychedelic sessions, optimizing clinical outcomes (Nutt et al., 2020).

### 10.3.3 Technological and Global Outlook

As clinical evidence accumulates, regulatory landscapes continue to shift. Several countries and municipalities are exploring decriminalization or controlled medical frameworks for psychedelic substances (Doblin et al., 2019). Parallel to these policy changes, new technologies are refining how therapeutic sessions are delivered and measured.

- Telehealth Expansion: Virtual preparation and integration sessions can broaden access to MDMA-assisted therapy, particularly for patients in remote areas or those with mobility challenges (George & Engel, 2021).
- Virtual Reality (VR) and Augmented Reality (AR): Early pilots suggest VR or AR could aid exposure therapy for PTSD when combined with the empathogenic effects of MDMA (Feduccia & Mithoefer, 2018).
- Global Collaboration Networks: Online platforms allow researchers and clinicians worldwide to share real-time data, enhancing study replication and accelerating innovation (Carhart-Harris & Goodwin, 2017).

## Conclusion

The Psychedelic Therapeutics Series will continue to evolve in tandem with the expanding scientific, cultural, and technological landscape of MDMA research. Building on the profound insights and therapeutic breakthroughs covered in this volume, subsequent entries may focus on mescaline, DMT, 5-MeO-DMT, or novel analogs of MDMA, each bringing unique therapeutic possibilities and challenges. As regulatory bodies and mainstream psychiatry begin to embrace the transformative potential of these agents, interdisciplinary collaborations and technological advances will play a central role in refining best practices and broadening patient access (Nutt et al., 2020).

## References


- Carhart-Harris, R. L., & Goodwin, G. M. (2017). The therapeutic potential of psychedelic drugs: Past, present, and future. Neuropsychopharmacology, 42(11), 2105–2113.
- Carhart-Harris, R. L., Roseman, L., Bolstridge, M., et al. (2018). Psychedelics and the essential importance of context. Journal of Psychopharmacology, 32(7), 725–731.
- de la Torre, R., Farré, M., & Torrens, M. (2020). MDMA analogs as potential treatments for psychiatric disorders: An update on pharmacology and clinical research. Pharmacology & Therapeutics, 208, 107483.
- Doblin, R., Christiansen, M., Jerome, I., & Burge, B. (2019). The past and future of MDMA-assisted psychotherapy for PTSD. Journal of Psychopharmacology, 33(12), 1180–1187.
- Feduccia, A. A., & Mithoefer, M. C. (2018). MDMA-assisted psychotherapy for PTSD: Are memory reconsolidation and fear extinction underlying mechanisms? Progress in Neuro-Psychopharmacology & Biological Psychiatry, 84, 221–228.
- George, S. A., & Engel, B. (2021). Telehealth and psychedelic-assisted therapies: Expanding accessibility and improving patient outcomes. Frontiers in Psychiatry, 12, 784511.
- González, D., Riba, J., & Barbanoj, M. (2022). Mescaline research in

clinical contexts: Past lessons and future prospects. Current Drug Abuse Reviews, 15(2), 99–110.

- Johnson, M. W., & Griffiths, R. R. (2017). Potential therapeutic effects of psilocybin. Neurotherapeutics, 14(3), 734–740.
- Nichols, D. E. (2016). Psychedelics. Pharmacological Reviews, 68(2), 264–355.
- Nutt, D., Erritzoe, D., & Carhart-Harris, R. (2020). Psychedelic psychiatry's brave new world. Cell, 181(1), 24–28.
- Sessa, B. (2017). MDMA therapy in the UK: A coming of age for psychedelic medicine. Journal of Psychoactive Drugs, 49(5), 427–432.

# About the Author

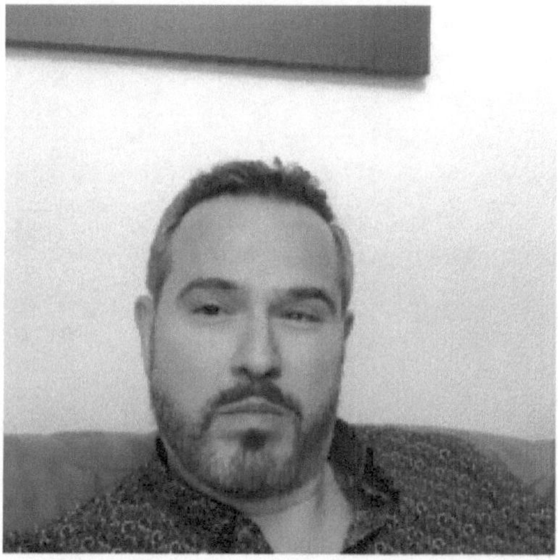

Dr. Nikolaos Tsilikas, of Greek origin, is a psychiatrist based in Switzerland with about 16 years of professional experience in the country. He earned his medical diploma in Greece and completed his FMH specialization in psychiatry in Switzerland in 2020.

He has worked extensively in Swiss public psychiatric institutions, including ambulatory services and hospitals, focusing on adult and geriatric psychiatry. Since late 2022, he has been running his private psychiatric practice in Neuchâtel, providing personalized care to adults and elderly patients.

His expertise and commitment to advancing mental health care have sparked his curiosity to learn about the therapeutic potential of psychedelics, offering a unique perspective at the intersection of psychiatry and emerging treatments.

Read more at Dr. Nikolaos Tsilikas' at **linkedin.com/in/nikolaostsilikas**[1].

1. **https://www.linkedin.com/in/nikolaostsilikas**

## Don't miss out!

Visit the website below and you can sign up to receive emails whenever Dr. Nikolaos Tsilikas publishes a new book. There's no charge and no obligation.

https://books2read.com/r/B-A-TDVFD-KWXWF

BOOKS 2 READ

Connecting independent readers to independent writers.

# Also by Dr. Nikolaos Tsilikas

**Psychedelic Therapeutics Series**
Psychedelic Therapeutics: A Comprehensive Guide to Psilocybin
Psychedelic Therapeutics: A Comprehensive Guide to LSD
Psychedelic Therapeutics: A Comprehensive Guide to MDMA

Watch for more at https://www.linkedin.com/in/nikolaostsilikas/.

www.ingramcontent.com/pod-product-compliance
Lightning Source LLC
LaVergne TN
LVHW090412210926
848480LV00002B/540